CONTRIBUTORS

James Robert Alberts, MD
Clinical Instructor
Orthopaedic Surgery
University of California, San Diego
San Diego, California

Carlo Bellabarba, MD
Assistant Professor
Department of Orthopaedic Surgery
Harborview Medical Center
University of Washington
Seattle, Washington

Nitin N. Bhatia, MD
Spine Surgery Fellow
Department of Orthopaedics and Rehabilitation
University of Miami School of Medicine
Jackson Memorial Hospital
Miami, Florida

Christopher M. Bono, MD
Assistant Professor of Orthopaedic Surgery
Boston University Medical Center
Boston, Massachusetts

Jens R. Chapman, MD
Professor
Departments of Orthopaedic Surgery
and Neurological Surgery
Harborview Medical Center
University of Washington
Seattle, Washington

Raman Dhawan, MD
Department of Orthopaedic Surgery
State University of New York
Upstate Medical University
Syracuse, New York

Pedro J. Díaz-Marchán, MD
Chief of Neuroradiology, Ben Taub General Hospital
Associate Professor Neuroradiology
Radiology Department
Baylor College of Medicine
Houston, Texas

William H. Donovan, MD
Professor and Chairman
Department of Physical Medicine and Rehabilitation
University of Texas Health Science Center at Houston
Houston, Texas

Nabil A. Ebraheim, MD
Medical College of Ohio
Department of Orthopaedics

Matthew D. Eichenbaum, MD
Spine Research Fellow
Department of Orthopaedic Surgery
Thomas Jefferson University Hospital and
The Rothman Institute
Philadelphia, Pennsylvania

Frank J. Eismont, MD
Co-Chairman, Department of Orthopedic Surgery
Professor of Orthopedic Surgery
University of Miami School of Medicine
Miami, Florida

Laurence N. Fitzhenry, MD
Spine Research Fellow
Department of Orthopaedic Surgery
The Rothman Institute
Philadelphia, Pennsylvania

Bruce E. Fredrickson, MD
Syracuse, New York

CONTRIBUTORS (CONT.)

Steven R. Garfin, MD
Professor and Chair
Department of Orthopaedic Surgery
University of California, San Diego
San Diego, California

Stanley D. Gertzbein, MD, FRCSC
Professor of Orthopedics
Department of Orthopedics
Baylor College of Medicine
Houston, Texas

Zbigniew Gugala, MD, PhD
Department of Orthopaedic Surgery
Baylor College of Medicine
Houston, Texas

Mitchell B. Harris, MD, FACS
Associate Professor
Department of Orthopaedic Surgery
Chief of Orthopaedic Trauma
Brigham and Women's Hospital
Harvard Medical School
Boston, Massachusetts

Michael H. Heggeness, MD
Professor of Orthopaedic Surgery
The Methodist Hospital
Houston, Texas

John A. Hipp, PhD
Director, Spine Research
Orthopedic Surgery
Baylor College of Medicine
Houston, Texas

Juan M. Latorre, MD
Spinal Cord Injury Fellow
Spinal Cord Injury Service Department
The Institute for Rehabilitation and Research
Houston, Texas

Ronald W. Lindsey, MD
Professor of Orthopaedic Surgery
Department of Orthopaedic Surgery
Baylor College of Medicine
Houston, Texas

Sohail K. Mirza, MD
Associate Professor
Departments of Orthopaedic Surgery and
Neurological Surgery
Harborview Medical Center
University of Washington
Seattle, Washington

Charles A. Reitman, MD
Assistant Professor
Department of Orthopedic Surgery
Baylor College of Medicine
Houston, Texas

Kern Singh, MD
Department of Orthopaedic Surgery
Rush-Presbyterian St. Luke's Medical Center
Chicago, Illinois

Alexander R. Vaccaro, MD
Professor
Department of Orthopaedic Surgery
The Rothman Institute
Philadelphia, Pennsylvania

Hansen A. Yuan, MD
Professor, Department of Orthopaedic and
Neurological Surgery
State University of New York
Upstate Medical University
Syracuse, New York

MANAGEMENT OF THORACOLUMBAR FRACTURES

EDITED BY
CHARLES A. REITMAN, MD
DEPARTMENT OF ORTHOPAEDIC SURGERY
BAYLOR COLLEGE OF MEDICINE
HOUSTON, TEXAS

SERIES EDITOR
THOMAS R. JOHNSON, MD
ORTHOPAEDIC SURGEONS, PSC
BILLINGS, MONTANA

American Academy of Orthopaedic Surgeons

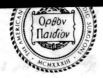
American Academy of Orthopaedic Surgeons
6300 North River Road
Rosemont, IL 60018
1-800-626-6726

The material presented in *Management of Thoracolumbar Fractures* has been made available by the American Academy of Orthopaedic Surgeons for educational purposes only. This material is not intended to present the only, or necessarily best, methods or procedures for the medical situations discussed, but rather is intended to represent an approach, view, statement, or opinion of the author(s) or producer(s), which may be helpful to others who face similar situations.

Some drugs or medical devices demonstrated in Academy courses or described in Academy print or electronic publications have not been cleared by the Food and Drug Administration (FDA) or have been cleared for specific uses only. The FDA has stated that it is the responsibility of the physician to determine the FDA clearance status of each drug or device he or she wishes to use in clinical practice.

The U.S. FDA has expressed concern about potential serious patient care issues involved with the use of polymethylmethacrylate (PMMA) bone cement in the spine. A physician might insert the PMMA bone cement into vertebrae by various procedures, including vertebroplasty and kyphoplasty.

PMMA bone cement is considered a device for FDA purposes. In October 1999, the FDA reclassified PMMA bone cement as a Class II device for its intended use "in arthroplastic procedures of the hip, knee, and other joints for the fixation of polymer or metallic prosthetic implants to living bone." The use of a device for other than its FDA-cleared indication is an off-label use. Physicians may use a device off-label if they believe, in their best medical judgment, that its use is appropriate for a particular patient (eg, tumors).

The use of PMMA bone cement in the spine is described in Academy educational courses, videotapes, and publications for educational purposes only. As is the Academy's policy regarding all of its educational offerings, the fact that the use of PMMA bone cement in the spine is discussed does not constitute an Academy endorsement of this use.

Furthermore, any statements about commercial products are solely the opinion(s) of the author(s) and do not represent an Academy endorsement or evaluation of these products. These statements may not be used in advertising or for any commercial purpose.

First Edition
Copyright © 2004 by the
American Academy of Orthopaedic Surgeons

ISBN 0-89203-322-3

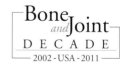

CONTENTS

CONTENTS (CONT.)

PREFACE

The annual incidence of spine fractures in the United States exceeds 150,000; young people continue to be principally affected, but injuries can occur in any age group. The thoracolumbar region is the most common site of vertebral fractures, second only to the cervical spine for fractures involving spinal cord injury. Thus, understanding how to manage these fractures is very important for anyone who cares for trauma patients. Because these injuries are so common, we have focused our discussion in this monograph on "true" thoracolumbar fractures, that is, those that occur from approximately T10 to L2.

Thoracolumbar fractures frequently occur as a result of high-energy mechanisms, most commonly motor vehicle accidents, followed by falls, gunshot wounds, and sports injuries; in this context, these fractures are evaluated as part of a multiple trauma injury assessment. Rapid assessment and progression through the emergency department is critical. Physical examination and indications for imaging studies are described in chapter 4. Delivery of oxygen and maintenance of blood pressure and body temperature are of paramount importance in initial management, as is provisional stabilization of the spine. In the presence of a neurologic deficit, pharmacologic agents such as high-dose methylprednisolone are often administered but remain controversial at this time, as discussed in detail in chapter 12. Of equal importance is early recognition of injuries to other body systems. In addition to noncontiguous spine injuries, fractures to the chest, long bones, and pelvis are common, as are intra-abdominal visceral injuries. Prompt recognition of injury patterns and understanding of their natural history are vital to appropriate management and decision making to optimize recovery and outcomes.

Unfortunately, despite the common occurrence of these injuries, many points of contention remain in approaches to management. A firm grasp of the mechanism of injury is essential to proceed with suitable care. For patients with spinal cord injuries, multiple body systems must be systematically evaluated and treated on an ongoing basis. Regardless of whether the patient has some degree of neurologic deficit, early mobilization is crucial whenever possible. It is important to recognize that most thoracolumbar injuries can be managed nonsurgically in patients with a favorable natural history.

Surgical indications generally involve decisions regarding stability. In many cases what exactly constitutes stability is highly controversial. As John A. Hipp, PhD, discusses in his chapter, several biomechanical studies have attempted to clarify the concepts of stability and evaluate stabilization procedures. Understanding in this area continues to evolve. Options for surgical fixation have increased and improved with the substantial growth in versatility of implants as discussed in chapter 7. Other challenges remain. Should I do surgery at all? What levels should I fuse? Should I decompress directly, indirectly, or is decompression necessary at all? Should I go in back, in front, in front from the back, or front and back? At times, the decision is clear, but frequently the answers are ambiguous. These concepts are well addressed in this monograph.

Rehabilitation is an essential component of recovery and return to work and society. Complications are inevitable and are certainly more prevalent in patients with traumatic injuries than in those undergoing elective surgery. Some complications develop as a result of the injury itself while others are problems associated with surgery. Continued vigilance in ongoing patient assessment is necessary to minimize, as well as facilitate correction of, complications.

Management of these fractures continues to be an evolving area of spine surgery and research. Methods to improve assessment and provide stability, as well as improve pharmacologic intervention, are currently being investigated and implemented. Care provided by emergency delivery systems, high-level trauma centers, and spinal injury centers has improved considerably, resulting in fewer complete spinal cord injuries, fewer acute care complications, and even decreased mortality. These improvements in outcomes have advanced the concepts of multidisciplinary interaction and care of these patients.

This monograph represents the cooperative effort of many people. I was very fortunate to enlist the help of a superb group of contributors. I am indebted to them, not only for what they have written but also for their willingness to be selfless educators. I would also like to thank the American Academy of Orthopaedic Surgeons for their faith and the opportunity to edit this monograph. I am particularly grateful for the steady assistance of Lynne Shindoll, Managing Editor, and Joan Abern, Senior Editor, both of whom believed in this project and helped make this monograph a reality. The entire staff of the Publications Department is to be congratulated for their insistence on producing the highest quality publications. Finally, I would like to thank my assistant, Kathy Wagner, for her endless help and support.

In everyone's life, there is a group of people who must be acknowledged, for they make you who you are. It is with great respect and honor that I first acknowledge my parents, Nan and Robert Reitman, the only role models I've ever had or needed. I would also like to thank Stephen Esses, my first mentor, who graciously guided me and gave me early opportunities to progress in this field. I also thank Ron Lindsey who encouraged me to proceed with this project. And finally, to Mychal, Matthew, Laura, and Allison, my children, and to Alicia, simply the best wife anyone ever had.

This monograph does not give you a recipe for treating thoracolumbar fractures. It does, however, thoroughly present the concepts that allow you to think and to treat patients in a thoughtful, well-considered fashion. I hope you enjoy reading this monograph as much as I did editing it.

Charles A. Reitman, MD

CHAPTER 1

SURGICAL ANATOMY OF THE THORACOLUMBAR SPINE

NABIL A. EBRAHEIM, MD
RONGMING XU, MD

The thoracolumbar junction is the most commonly injured area of the spine. A thorough knowledge of the surgical anatomy of the thoracolumbar spine is necessary for optimal management of spinal injuries and to avoid or minimize surgical complications. This chapter reviews the basic anatomy of the thoracolumbar spine, including the bony structures, articulations, ligaments, neural structures, blood supply, and musculature.

BONY STRUCTURES

The basic components of the vertebrae of the thoracolumbar spine are the vertebral body, the overall dimensions of which gradually decrease from the thoracic to the lumbar spine, and the neural arch. The neural arch is composed of the pedicles, situated laterally, and the laminae, located posteriorly. The pedicles, which connect the vertebral body with the laminae, are short tubular structures and are the strongest portion of the vertebrae. Adjacent pedicles form the superior and inferior borders of the intervertebral foramen. The spinous process is posterior to the fusion of the laminae. The spinous process increases in size from the thoracic to the lumbar region. Lateral to the junction of the pedicle and the lamina is the transverse process. The superior articular processes, on which the facet surface is directly posterior, project from the upper border of each lamina. The inferior articular processes, on which the facet surface is directly anterior, project from the caudal portion of each lamina.

THE THORACIC VERTEBRAE

The structures unique to the thoracic vertebral bodies (Figure 1) are the facets that are located on the upper and lower portions of the lateral surface of the vertebral body and articulate with the rib head, forming the costovertebral joint. The thoracic pedicle projects posteriorly from the upper portion of the vertebral body; its superoinferior diameter is larger than the mediolateral diameter. The mean pedicle widths and heights for vertebrae T1 through T12 vary from approximately 4 to 10 mm and from 8 to 17 mm, respectively.[1-3] The midthoracic pedicles are the smallest, and the lower thoracic pedicles are the largest. The thickest wall of the thoracic pedicle is the medial wall.[4] The projection point of the pedicle axis is located medial to the lateral edge of the superior facet and superior to the midline of the transverse process, which is the ideal entrance for pedicle screw insertion (Figure 2). In general, the medial inclination of the pedicle decreases from T1 to T12. The superior and inferior facets arise from the upper and lower part of the pedicle of the thoracic vertebrae. The superior facet lies cranially, with the articular surface on the dorsal aspect; the inferior facet lies caudally, with the articular surface toward the ventral aspect. The facet joint of a thoracic vertebra is quite different from that of the cervical and lumbar vertebrae because it is oriented more in the coronal plane. This plays an important role in the stabilization of the thoracic spine during flexion loading because the anterior translation of the thoracic vertebrae is limited by the facet joints.

FIGURE 1

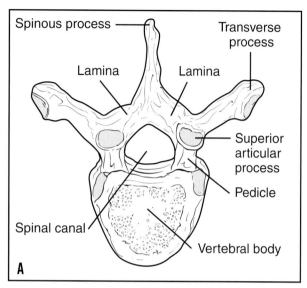

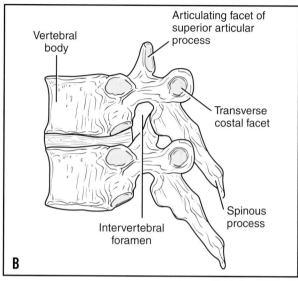

A, Superior view of thoracic vertebra. **B,** Lateral view of thoracic vertebrae.

FIGURE 2

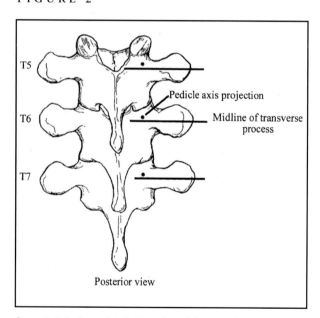

Suggested starting points for thoracic pedicle screws based on the center of the pedicle axis.

Viewing the spine posteriorly, the neural arch below the level of the transverse process can be divided into two portions; a medial half for the lamina and a lateral half for the inferior articular process (Figure 3). The laminar width is approximately 9 to 10 mm for vertebrae T1 through T12.[5]

THE LUMBAR VERTEBRAE

The lumbar vertebrae are larger and heavier than the thoracic vertebrae (Figure 4). When viewed superiorly, the vertebral body appears kidney shaped. The spinal canal is triangular, most distinctly at L5. The angled lateral borders of the spinal canal, called the lateral recesses, constitute the bony canal of the spinal nerve root. The pedicles are short and have a slight medial inclination. In general, the pedicle width increases gradually from L1 to L5; pedicle height varies among individuals.[1,6,7] The pedicle lengths measured between the dorsal and ventral cortex of the vertebra average 40 to 50 mm, and the medial inclination of the pedicle increases consistently from L1 to L5. The projection point of the pedicle axis is located above the midline of the transverse process at the levels above L4 (Figure 5). At L4, the projection point is close to the midline of the transverse process. At L5, this point is located inferior to the midline of the transverse process.[6]

The laminae of the lumbar vertebrae are thicker and oriented in a more vertical direction in the sagittal plane than the laminae of the thoracic vertebrae. The portion of the lamina between the superior and inferior articular processes and just below the level of the pedicle is the isthmus or pars interarticularis, which is a common site of stress fractures. The superior and inferior articular facets are also quite different from those in the thoracic region, which are oriented in the sagittal plane. The superior articular surface is concave and faces posteromedially, whereas the inferior articular surface is convex and faces anterolaterally. The facet angles relative to the sagittal plane range from 120° to 150°, decreasing consistently from L1 to L5.[8,9]

ARTICULATIONS

Articulations are present between vertebrae and include the intervertebral disk anteriorly and the facet, or zygapophyseal, joints posteriorly. These articulations are reinforced by ligaments.

The intervertebral disks are located between adjacent vertebral bodies and allow flexion, extension, and lateral bending motion. They consist mainly of the nucleus pulposus, located in the central portion; the anulus fibrosus, located in the outer portion; and cartilaginous end plates adjacent to the surfaces of the vertebral bodies. The nucleus pulposus is composed mainly of mucoid material that is 70% to 90% water.[10] The anulus fibrosus, which consists of collagenous fibers, looks like a laminated structure surrounding the nucleus pulposus. The posterior portion of the anulus fibrosus is thinner than the anterior portion. The fibers of the lamellae are arranged in a

FIGURE 3

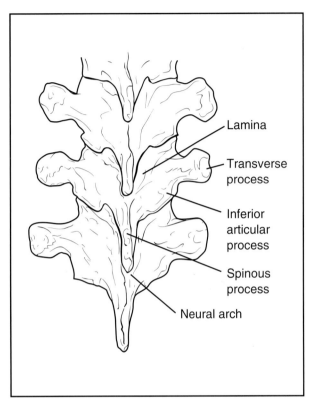

Posterior view of the thoracic spine showing the lamina (medial half) and the inferior articular process.

FIGURE 4

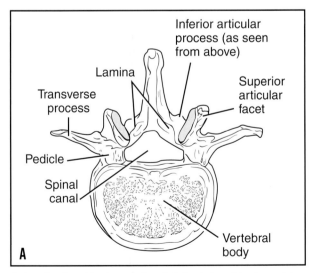

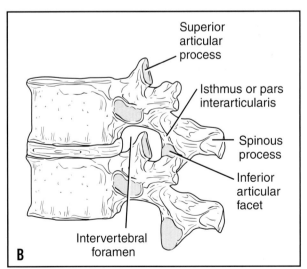

A, Superior view of lumbar vertebra. **B,** Lateral view of lumbar vertebrae.

FIGURE 5

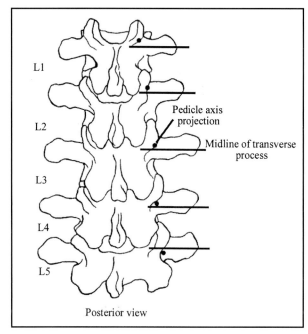

Suggested starting points for lumbar pedicle screws based on the center of the pedicle axis.

FIGURE 6

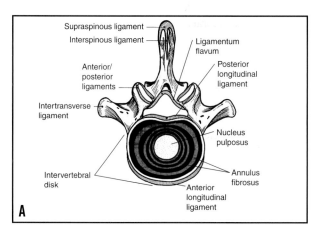

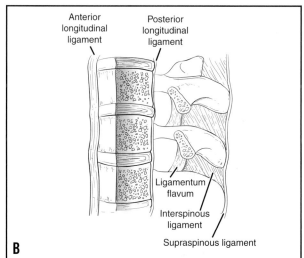

Superior (A) and lateral (B) views of the ligaments in the thoracolumbar spine.

concentric oblique direction and overlap one another. The cartilaginous end plate is the layer located between the vertebral body and the disk, which functions as a growth plate and facilitates the transfer of nutrients from the vertebral body to the disk.

The facet joint is a synovial joint that consists of the adjacent inferior and superior articular processes and the articular capsule. The articular surfaces are covered by hyaline cartilage, which allows sliding motion to occur in the posterior arch of the spinal column. The articular capsules are thin and have an inner synovial membrane and an outer fibrous membrane. They attach peripherally to the articular surfaces of the facet joints.

LIGAMENTS

Several ligaments play an important role in stabilizing the thoracolumbar spine as one unit (Figure 6). These include the anterior and posterior longitudinal ligaments; the ligamentum flava, or yellow ligaments; and the supraspinous and interspinous ligaments.

The anterior longitudinal ligament is a strong band

that attaches to the entire anterior aspect of the vertebral bodies and intervertebral disks. It is thicker anteriorly and thinner laterally. The most superficial fibers are the longest, extending over three or four vertebrae. The deepest fibers extend over two vertebrae and are firmly attached from the inferior margin of one vertebra to the superior margin of the next. The main function of the anterior longitudinal ligament is to limit extension of the spinal column.

The posterior longitudinal ligament attaches to the posterior aspect of the vertebral bodies and disks. In the thoracic and lumbar regions, this ligament is narrow over the middle of the vertebrae and broad over the disks. As with the anterior longitudinal ligament, the superficial fibers of the posterior longitudinal ligament extend over three or four vertebrae, and the deeper fibers bridge only adjacent vertebrae. The role of the posterior longitudinal ligament is to stabilize the spinal column during flexion.

The ligamentum flava are located between the laminae of adjacent vertebrae; they join together in the midline. They are composed mainly of yellow elastic fibers that run vertically. Each ligamentum flavum attaches to the lower portion of the anterior surface of the upper lamina and the upper portion of the posterior surface of the lower lamina, covering the entire interlaminar space.[11-13] Laterally, the ligamentum flavum fuses with the capsule of the facet joint. In the lumbar spine, the ligamentum flavum is very thick.

The interspinous and supraspinous ligaments connect the spinous processes posteriorly. The interspinous ligament is thin. The supraspinous ligament is thicker and stronger and extends over the spinous processes.

NEURAL STRUCTURES

The neural structures of the thoracolumbar spine are shown in Figure 7. The spinal cord ends between T12-L1 and L2-3.[14] The end of the spinal cord is called the conus medullaris and becomes a bundle of nerve roots termed the cauda equina. The spinal cord enlarges between L1 and S3.

The spinal nerves exit along the spinal canal. In the thoracic spine, these nerves lie in the middle of the intervertebral foramina. In the lumbar spine, they lie in the upper portion of the foramina.[15,16] In the lumbar spine, the spinal nerves are close to the medioinferior border of the upper pedicle.[14,17] Most ganglia of the thoracic and lumbar spinal nerves lie within the intervertebral foramen.[14,18,19]

After exiting from the intervertebral foramina, each spinal nerve divides into a small dorsal ramus and a large ventral ramus. The dorsal rami course posteriorly to supply the spinal ligaments and the muscles and skin of the back. The ventral rami are longer and run laterally in the thoracic region and lateroinferiorly in the lumbar region.

BLOOD SUPPLY

The arterial blood supply to the spine is shown in Figure 8. Paired intercostal and lumbar arteries, originating directly from the thoracic and abdominal aorta, supply

FIGURE 7

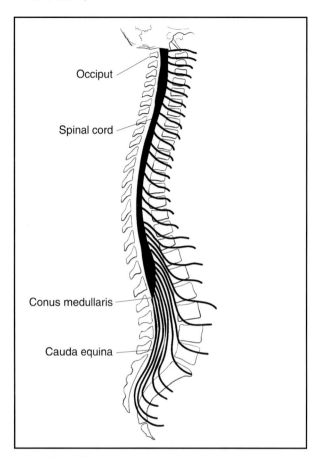

Lateral view of the spinal cord and cauda equina.

the thoracic and lumbar spine. The main blood supply to the spinal cord consists of a single anterior spinal artery, paired posterior spinal arteries, and several radicular (medullary) arteries. The number of medullary arteries varies from the cervical to lumbar region because only a few segmental arteries branch off the medullary arteries to join with the anterior spinal artery.[20] The lower thoracic and lumbosacral cord regions are usually supplied by either one or three medullary arteries.[21] The most caudal medullary artery of the spine, also called Adamkiewicz' artery, is the largest, with a mean diameter of 0.9 mm. It usually originates from the lower intercostal or upper lumbar artery.[22] The medullary arteries provide a vital blood supply to the anterior spinal artery. The spinal cord may be at risk of ischemia if the anterior spinal artery is compromised by disk herniation or frac-

FIGURE 8

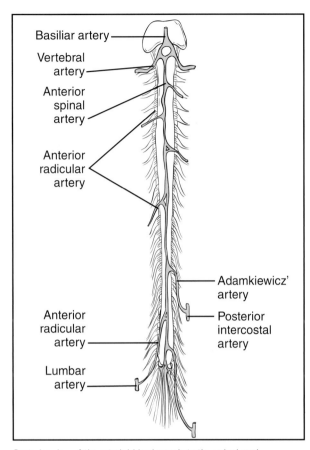

Basiliar artery

Vertebral artery

Anterior spinal artery

Anterior radicular artery

Anterior radicular artery

Lumbar artery

Adamkiewicz' artery

Posterior intercostal artery

Posterior view of the arterial blood supply to the spinal cord.

ture or if the medullary artery is injured. In some patients, the radicular arteries also supply blood to the cauda equina.[23,24]

Veins surrounding the spinal cord include an anterior internal vertebral venous plexus and a posterior internal vertebral venous plexus. These are valveless venous structures in the epidural space.

MUSCULATURE

In the thoracolumbar region, the superficial muscle is the latissimus dorsi, which covers the entire lower half of the back. It arises from the posterior layer of the thoracolumbar fascia and inserts into the intertubercular groove of the humerus. The posterior layer of the thoracolumbar fascia is thin in the thoracic region but thick and strong in the lumbar region; this morphology may play an

important role in rotation of the trunk and stabilization of the lower back.[25] The intermediate layer of the posterior muscles of the spine includes the splenius and serratus. The deep layer of the posterior muscle consists of the erector spinae muscles, which are vertically oriented muscle bundles that extend from the iliocrosolumbar region up to the cervical region. Three distinct columns comprise the erector spinae muscles under the thoracolumbar fascia in the lumbar region: the iliocostalis laterally, the longissimus centrally, and the spinalis medially. The functions of the most posterior muscles of the spine include extension, lateral bending, and rotation of the spine. The lateral or anterolateral muscles of the spine in the lumbar region include the iliopsoas major and the quadratus lumborum. Most of these muscles contribute to flexion and rotation of the spine.

SUMMARY AND CONCLUSIONS

The basic anatomy of the thoracolumbar spine has been described in this chapter. Internal fixation of the thoracolumbar spine, regardless of the technique used, carries a risk of injury to the adjacent vital structures. Therefore, the surgeon should be thoroughly familiar with the three-dimensional anatomy of the thoracolumbar spine to minimize surgical complications. In addition, because of anatomic variations that occur among individuals, preoperative imaging studies should be obtained routinely.

REFERENCES

1. Zindrick MR, Wiltse LL, Doornik A: Analysis of the morphometric characteristics of the thoracic and lumbar pedicles. *Spine* 1987;12:160-166.
2. Panjabi MM, Takata K, Geol V, et al: Thoracic human vertebrae: Quantitative three-dimensional anatomy. *Spine* 1991;16:888-901.
3. Ebraheim NA, Xu R, Ahmad M, Yeasting RA: Projection of the thoracic pedicle and its morphometric analysis. *Spine* 1997;22:233-238.
4. Kothe R, O'Holleran JD, Liu W, Panjabi MM: Internal architecture of the thoracic pedicle. *Spine* 1996;21:264-270.
5. Ebraheim NA, Xu R, Ahmad M, Yeasting RA: The quantitative anatomy of the thoracic facet and the posterior projection of its inferior facet. *Spine* 1997;22:1811-1818.
6. Ebraheim NA, Rollins JR, Xu R, Yeasting RA: Projection of the lumbar pedicle and its morphometric analysis. *Spine* 1996;21:1296-1300.

7. Panjabi MM, Goel V, Oxland T, et al: Human lumbar vertebrae: Quantitative three-dimensional anatomy. *Spine* 1992;17:299-306.

8. Panjabi MM, Oxland T, Takata K, et al: Articular facets of the human spine. *Spine* 1993;18:1298-1310.

9. Van-Schaik JPJ, Verbiest H, Van-Schaik FDJ: The orientation of laminae and facet joints in the lower lumbar spine. *Spine* 1985;10:59-63.

10. Bogduk N, Twomey LT: The inter-body joints and the intervertebral discs, in Bogduk N, Twomey LT (eds): *Clinical Anatomy of the Lumbar Spine,* ed 2. Edinburgh, Scotland, Churchill Livingstone, 1991, pp 11-26.

11. Olszewski AD, Yaszemski MJ, White AA: The anatomy of the human lumbar ligamentum flavum. *Spine* 1996;21:2307-2312.

12. Ramsey RH: The anatomy of the ligamenta flava. *Clin Orthop* 1966;44:129-140.

13. Yong-Hing K, Reilly J, Kirkaldy-Willis WH: The ligamentum flavum. *Spine* 1976;1:226-234.

14. Louis R: Topographic relationships of the vertebral column, spinal cord, and nerve roots. *Anat Clin* 1978;1:3-12.

15. Ebraheim NA, Jabaly G, Xu R, Yeasting RA: Anatomic relations of the thoracic pedicle to the adjacent neural structures. *Spine* 1997;22:1553-1557.

16. Rauschining W: Normal and pathologic anatomy of the lumbar root canals. *Spine* 1987;12:1008-1019.

17. Ebraheim NA, Xu R, Darwich M, Yeasting RA: Anatomic relations between the lumbar pedicle and the adjacent neural structures. *Spine* 1997;22:2338-2341.

18. Cohen MS, Wall EJ, Brown RA, Rydevik B, Garfin SR: Cauda equina anatomy II: Extrathecal nerve roots and dorsal root ganglia. *Spine* 1990;15:1248-1251.

19. Hasegawa T, Mikawa Y, Watanabe R, An HS: Morphometric analysis of the lumbosacral nerve roots and dorsal root ganglia by magnetic resonance imaging. *Spine* 1996;21:1005-1009.

20. Dommisse GF: The blood supply of the spinal cord. *J Bone Joint Surg Br* 1974;56:225-235.

21. Schoenen J: Clinical anatomy of the spinal cord, in Young RR, Woolsey RM (eds): *Diagnosis and Management of Disorders of the Spinal Cord.* Philadelphia, PA, WB Saunders, 1995, pp 1-28.

22. Lu J, Ebraheim NA, Biyani A, Brown JA, Yeasting RA: Vulnerability of great medullary artery. *Spine* 1996;21:1852-1855.

23. Dommisse GF, Grobler L: Arteries and veins of the lumbar nerve roots and cauda equina. *Clin Orthop* 1976;115:22-29.

24. Parke WW, Gammell K, Rothman RH: Arterial vascularization of the cauda equina. *J Bone Joint Surg Am* 1981;63:53-62.

25. Vleeming A, Pool-Goudzwaard AL, Stoeckart R, Van-Wingerden J, Snijders CJ: The posterior layer of the thoracolumbar fascia. *Spine* 1995;20:753-758.

CHAPTER 2

BIOMECHANICS OF THORACOLUMBAR FRACTURES

JOHN A. HIPP, PHD

The primary goal in treating thoracolumbar fractures is to optimize the final outcome, striving to achieve the fastest, most complete restoration of function and anatomy. Understanding the biomechanics of these fractures plays an important role in achieving this goal. The initial steps include estimating the loads that caused the injury, assessing the damages using noninvasive imaging, and compiling that information within the framework provided by research into the biomechanics of spinal fractures. Once the damage is identified and its effect on the mechanical functions of the spine is estimated, this knowledge is then used to help select the optimal treatment. Although the method of treatment depends on many factors, from a biomechanical perspective, the best treatment can be selected with support from biomechanical tests of different types of fixation.

OVERVIEW OF RESEARCH FINDINGS

What Is Known

The bulk of the research has been done on cervical and lower lumbar fractures, and because some biomechanical principles are common to the entire spine, the results of this research can help in understanding fracture mechanisms and the biomechanics of treatment of thoracolumbar frac-

tures. In addition, several excellent biomechanical studies have been completed that specifically address thoracolumbar fractures and treatment. It is known that the thoracic spine is relatively stiff compared with other areas of the spine. The rib cage, thoracic musculature, and the articulations between the ribs and the spine are unique to the thoracic spine. In addition, the mechanical properties of the spine have been studied, including the properties of the intervertebral disks, the strength of the articulations between ribs and the spine, the load-bearing capacity of individual vertebrae, and the load-bearing capacity of complete segments of the spine. The amount of motion that normally occurs between vertebrae during various activities has been measured, as has the increase in motion that occurs when ligaments and articulations are sectioned during laboratory tests. The resulting data help clinicians identify abnormalities in motion, which in turn help identify damage to the spine. Finally, the ability of different types of fixation to mechanically stabilize the spine has been measured, and the many variables, such as bone density, that can affect the stability provided by fixation systems have been described.

What Is Not Known

For all that is known about thoracolumbar fractures, much is not known. Researchers have yet to achieve the ultimate goals of having (1) diagnostic tests that reliably and accurately document the exact soft-tissue and bony damage, (2) proven treatment guidelines that use the results of diagnostic tests to help select the optimal treatment, and (3) treatments that optimize the final outcome. Another major unknown is the mechanical goal of various internal fixation systems. Initially it was assumed that the best fixation system reduced intervertebral motion the most and created the stiffest construct. In fact, a small amount of motion may be desirable since this can encourage rapid bone formation and subsequent fusion. Unfortunately, it remains unknown how much motion is needed to encourage fracture healing or spinal fusion; thus, it is difficult to assess the results of biomechanical testing. In addition, the fixation system must not fail under the loads of activities of daily living. Although experimental models have been developed to predict the loads applied to the spine during some activities of daily living, consensus is lacking on how much load must be supported by the thoracolumbar spine both during and after healing of a thoracolumbar injury.

Determining the Damage

When the spine is subjected to excessive forces, it will fail. Exactly how it fails is determined by the direction, rate, and magnitude of the loads, as well as by the mechanical properties of each individual spine. Ultimate damage is estimated by analyzing information gathered from the history, physical examination, and imaging studies and combining it with known results from biomechanical experiments and computer models. This process is complicated by the fact that, during the actual trauma, very dramatic displacements can occur between vertebrae that may never be appreciated following the injury. Elasticity in the bone and soft tissues, as well as the stabilizing effect of the rib cage and thoracic musculature, can reduce many displacements that occur transiently during trauma. Transient retropulsion of bone into the canal, immediately followed by partial reduction of the fragment, has been demonstrated in laboratory tests.[1] In addition, spinal cord injury without radiologic abnormality has been described by several authors.[2] It has been suggested that any injury to the spine that results in a neurologic injury should be considered unstable. This is based on the hypothesis that any transient vertebral displacements that result in neurologic injury must be associated with damage to the disk and ligaments that normally prevent excessive displacements. This hypothesis has never been proven, although accepting this hypothesis may be the safest approach.

Various classification systems have been described for thoracolumbar fractures, based on common noninvasive imaging modalities.[3] A classification system should provide a means for easily describing an injury so that there is reliable communication among physicians. To achieve this goal, all clinicians must classify fractures consistently. The level of interobserver agreement achieved with two common classification systems (Denis and AO/Magerl) applied to both MRI and CT scans of clinical thoracolumbar fractures has been studied.[3] Overall, the authors found moderate agreement using these classification systems, although in several cases agreement between certain observers was poor, and in some cases, the classifications derived from the CT scans did not agree with the classifications made from the MRI scans. Thus, existing classification systems can be helpful, but this clinical efficacy has never been proved.

Knowledge of the specific soft-tissue and bony damage to the spine could be very useful in determining how to best repair the damage. The goal of identifying which ligaments are damaged and quantifying the stability of any bone fractures is challenging in light of a study where careful analysis of MRI scans showed large variations in the condition of the bone and soft tissues of patients with thoracolumbar fractures.[4] That study also failed to find any pattern between the MRI findings and a common classification system for these injuries, raising concerns about how much insight some of the current classification systems offer. Another investigation showed that, when carefully used, MRI can detect acute damage to the intervertebral disk.[5] However, in routine clinical practice, current diagnostic tests may only provide a general understanding of the actual damage to the spine and have never been proved to effectively aid in determining how best to treat a fracture.

Mechanism of Injury

The energy delivered to the spine and the magnitude and direction of forces that cause the injury determine which tissues are damaged; therefore, it is always important to identify the events that resulted in the fracture. Unfortunately, the sensitivity and specificity of identifying specific damage to the spine from the history of the injury has never been assessed. Nevertheless, the description of the injury event is commonly used to estimate the damage. In general, the bone injuries that may occur as a result of an injury to the spine are determined by the normal internal architecture of the vertebrae. Heggeness and Doherty[6] demonstrated that a trabecular framework exists within the vertebrae. Trabeculae run from the medial aspect of the pedicles, extending radially to the anterior and lateral aspects of the body. This radial orientation can account for the shape of fragments seen in burst fractures, where the edges of the fragments are coincident with the trabecular directions. The soft-tissue injuries are determined by the properties of the tissues, the strength of the attachment to bone, and the proportion of the load supported by each soft-tissue component. Soft-tissue injuries caused by specific types of loading have been reported, and it is helpful to understand the damage caused by simple types of loading.

Axial Loading

The normal kyphotic curvature of the thoracic spine makes it unlikely that the spine can be damaged by a purely compressive or tensile load. However, laboratory testing has shown that when pure compressive forces are applied to the spine, end plate fractures typically appear with lower forces, wedge fractures occur with intermediate loads, and burst fractures occur when the loads are high and fast enough.[7-10] If the vertebral body alone fails as a result of pure compressive force, the fracture tends to be stable, presumably the result of consolidation of the bone. In the fracture classification system of Denis, a fracture caused by up to 50% compression of the vertebral body (without posterior ligamentous damage) is considered to be a stable fracture. However, it is important to recognize that posterior ligamentous damage may be difficult to detect in the acute setting, and it is important to look for damage to the vertebral levels above and below the fracture.[11]

Higher energy trauma with axially directed loads results in burst fractures. Burst fractures created in a laboratory setting showed that motion segments were two times more flexible in flexion and extension, 2.7 times more flexible in lateral bending, and more than four times more flexible with tension/compression or axial rotation.[7] Additional studies showed that end plate fractures alone did not increase intervertebral motion enough to be clinically detectable, but wedge fractures significantly increased intervertebral motion in flexion and extension, lateral bending, and axial rotation. Burst fractures led to even more dramatic increases in instability.[12] However, in those laboratory studies, the measured intervertebral rotations were obtained in specimens dissected free of all surrounding musculature and the rib cage. In a clinical setting, the instability and reduced motion that might be

seen in a flexion–extension study following a burst fracture (if this test could be safely performed) might be much less pronounced because of the stabilizing effect of surrounding muscles and the rib cage and pain limitations or muscle spasms. Wang and associates,[13] in a study of experimentally created burst fractures, reported that intervertebral disks two levels below the fractured disk can be damaged as a result of the fracture, and this damage may not be detected on radiographs. Pure axial compressive loads can also damage the facet joints since a portion of the axial load is normally supported by the facets. This complex loading pattern through the facets can be transmitted to the remainder of the posterior elements, resulting in fractures of the lamina or pedicle. Once the posterior elements are fractured or the posterior ligaments are severely disrupted, fractures of the anterior vertebral body become very unstable because the tension band effect of the posterior structures is lost.

Flexion

Pure sagittal plane moments applied to the isolated spine create tensile forces in parts of the spine that are balanced by compressive forces in other parts of the spine. When a pure moment (not a superimposed axial load) is applied, there will be a neutral point with zero force at a particular point in the spine, with gradually increasing compressive forces on one side of neutral and gradually increasing tensile forces on the other side. If the neutral point is located immediately in front of the posterior longitudinal ligament during flexion, then flexion will result in compression of the anterior body and distraction of the posterior elements. This can disrupt the posterior ligaments and possibly fracture the anterior aspect of the vertebrae if the moments are high enough. If the neutral point of the flexion moment is located well in front of the vertebral body, as in a seat belt injury, then the entire spine can be loaded in tension. However, flexion is probably almost always combined with axial loads. When combined with a distractive load, the compressive component caused by the flexion moment will be reduced or replaced by tension and will dramatically increase tensile stresses on the posterior elements. This results in more severe avulsions, posterior bone fractures, and ligament damage. The spine generally is not subjected to tensile-type loads; therefore, it is not well adapted to resisting these loads.

Extension

When an extension moment is applied to the spine in the sagittal plane, tensile forces that occur in the anterior aspects of the spine must be balanced by compressive forces in the posterior aspect of the spine. Langrana and associates[14] offered evidence to support the hypothesis that high loads are transmitted through the facets when an extension moment is applied to the spine, especially when this moment is combined with axial compressive loading. This loading mode can actually create clinically realistic burst fractures. The data also suggest that loading of the facets creates shear forces that may contribute to retropulsion of bone fragments into the spinal canal.

Shear

The biomechanical consequences of pure shear-type loading have not been extensively studied in the laboratory. A shear type of load results in disruption of the intervertebral disk and the intervertebral ligaments, causing a very unstable spine. When pure shear loads are applied to the thoracolumbar spine, the resulting vertebral displacements include a flexion–extension component given the geometry of the facets and rib articulations. It is known that the facets play a very important role in resisting shear. It would be expected that for a pure shear type of loading, the facets and rib articulations would be damaged first, followed by other complex types of damage, including facet dislocations.

Axial Rotation

The rib cage and the articulations between the ribs and the spine play a very important role in determining the damage to the thoracic spine that is the result of axial rotation. The thoracic cage has a very large cross section compared with the isolated thoracic spine and can support the thoracic spine over a large moment arm. This arrangement can stabilize the spine and prevent injury. Conversely, if transverse forces are applied to the thoracic cage, the effect of the force can be magnified by the moment arm and contribute to an injury to the thoracic spine. Additionally, forces delivered at the thoracolumbar junction are further exaggerated by the fact that this junction represents an abrupt transition of the more rigid, stable thoracic portion to the more flexible lumbar portion of the spinal column. The facet joints also help control intervertebral motion during axial rotation. As much as 45% of torsional forces may be transmitted through the facet joints, and traumatic axial rotation can fracture the facets or disrupt the joint capsules. Either one or both of the facets can be fractured. Since the facets normally support a significant portion of axial rotation, facet fractures can result in substantial instability.

Combined Loading Mechanisms

The spine is rarely damaged by pure tensile, compressive, or bending-type loads. Damage usually is the result of a more complex type of combined loading. In addition, the interaction between the biomechanical properties of an individual spine and the effect that individual load components will have on a particular spine is very important. All pure loading modes are associated with some amount of coupled motion in the thoracic spine.[15] The interaction between the orientation of the spine and the direction of applied loads is also important. Even with simple compressive loads to the body, the actual forces on the spine can be complex. The fracture pattern caused by this compression depends on the flexion angle of the spine at the time of loading.[16] The load that is actually applied to a specific thoracolumbar vertebra when external loads are directed along the long axis of the body generally will be a combination of compression, shear, and bending. The magnitude of each load component depends on the position of the body at the time of the injury. Therefore, the position of the body relative to the direction and magnitude of the load should be considered when describing the mechanism of injury to estimate the damage to the spine. To make the issue even more confusing, in a retrospective clinical study, Hsu and associates[17] found no significant correlation between the reported mechanism of injury and the presence of a vertebral fracture.

SELECTING THE OPTIMAL TREATMENT

The overall goal of treatment is to achieve a good clinical result. From a mechanical viewpoint, the best treatment (1) restores alignment without causing further neurologic damage, (2) augments damaged sections of the spine so that loads associated with activities of daily living can pass safely through the damaged region, (3) minimizes relative motion between any fracture fragments so that they can heal, and (4) minimally disturbs adjacent segments to avoid accelerating degenerative changes. Each of these goals must be considered when selecting a treatment.

Normal Kyphosis of the Thoracolumbar Spine

The amount of normal kyphosis of the thoracic spine ranges widely based on measurements made in young, healthy subjects who have no back pain.[18] Measurements range between 7° and 63°, with over 90% of the population falling between 18° and 51°. Korovessis and associates[19] reported that thoracic kyphosis increases with age, but they found no evidence of a gender difference. However, threshold levels of thoracic kyphosis that are both sensitive and specific for injury have not been reported, although kyphosis outside of the published normal ranges should be noted. The published ranges for kyphosis are for the entire thoracic spine. Lack of continuity in the overall curve of the spine clearly indicates an injury, although no validated guidelines are yet available that allow specific measurements to be used to estimate the extent of damage.

Normal Spinal Canal and Foraminal Dimensions

One of the main functions of the spine is to protect the spinal cord, conus medullaris, cauda equina, and nerve roots; this is achieved in part by continuously providing a protected space for the neural elements. Therefore, any evidence that this protected space has been compromised by an injury is important. The normal dimensions of the canal are covered in other chapters of this monograph. The spinal canal or nerve root foramina can be compromised by retropulsed bone fragments, intervertebral disk herniations, and/or by posterior apophyseal ring fractures.[20] MRI and CT can be used to detect and characterize these mechanisms for canal compromise. There are no validated guidelines for determining how much canal compromise is acceptable, although any evidence of compromise is an important clinical finding. In a study of canal compromise, Mohanty and Venkatram[21] suggested that the extent of neurologic recovery does not depend on the apparent initial extent of canal compromise. Gertzbein[22] also reported only a weak correlation between the extent of canal compromise and the amount of neurologic deficit. Fontijne and associates[23] reported that although the severity of neurologic injury could not be predicted from the extent of canal compromise, they found a significant correlation between the extent of canal compromise and the existence of neurologic injury, with the strength of the correlation greatest in the upper thoracic region. Clearly several factors interact to determine whether a violation of the canal or foraminal space should be corrected.

Mechanical Instability

With respect to the mechanical functions of the spine, instability can be defined as the inability to support patient activities without excessive pain or loss of neurologic function or anatomic alignment. This definition is intended to specifically exclude conditions such as a fracture that will heal uneventfully and without loss of anatomic alignment or neurologic function, even though the fracture may cause pain during the initial period of weight bearing. The vertebral bodies, intervertebral disks, facet joints and capsules, rib articulations, the various intervertebral ligaments, the surrounding muscles, and the thoracic cage all play a role in stabilizing the spine. Damage to any one component can compromise stability, although these structures work together and each component can also assume additional mechanical demand to accommodate for damage to other components. Thus, assessing the stability of the spine and identifying specific structural damage responsible for any instability can be very challenging.

Normal and Abnormal Ranges of Motion Between Vertebrae

Overall, the thoracic spine normally allows for much less motion than either the cervical or lumbar spines. Between T1 and T6, flexion and extension results in only 4° of intervertebral rotation, with motion increasing from 5° at T6-T7 to 12° at T12-L1.[24] During a flexion–extension maneuver, the center of rotation between vertebrae is normally located within the posterior third of the vertebral bodies.[25] Damage to the posterior elements in particular can lead to large increases in intervertebral rotation during flexion.[26] Damage to the intervertebral disk can also lead to large increases in intervertebral motion.[27] In lateral bending, rotation between vertebrae is approximately 6° at all levels from T1 to T10. Between T10 and L1, the amount of intervertebral rotation increases to approximately 8° at each level. In a laboratory study, Oda and associates[26] showed that disruption of the costovertebral joints resulted in a large increase in intervertebral motion with lateral bending and axial rotation. When a patient twists in a side-to-side motion, the amount of axial rotation between vertebrae is approximately 8° from T1 to T8, then decreases to about 2° in the upper lumbar spine. This substantial reduction in motion at the lower thoracic spine is primarily the result of the geometry of the facet joints, which facilitate axial rotation in the upper thoracic spine and impede axial rotation in the lower thoracic spine. It should also be noted that the thoracic spine is least flexible under axial loading.[15] The junction between the thoracic and lumbar spine is unique, in part because of the relatively sudden increase in intervertebral motion that occurs about this junction.

In clinical practice, it is not known if there are threshold levels of intervertebral motion that can be used to determine if there was soft-tissue or skeletal damage at a particular level. Nevertheless, intervertebral motion that occurs outside of normal limits should be noted and considered a possible indicator of instability. In a laboratory study, where known forces were applied to produce flexion and extension of the spine, Panjabi and associates[28] reported that only about 1 mm of shear normally occurs between thoracic vertebrae, and at failure, horizontal translation of one vertebra over the other is approximately 2.5 mm. The authors suggest that a static horizontal displacement of more than 2.5 mm may indicate failure and therefore an unstable spine. They also assert that the articulations between the ribs and the vertebrae are very important to the mechanical stability of the thoracic spine, suggesting that damage to these articulations may destabilize the spine. Other investigators have shown in the laboratory that intervertebral motion increases after the posterior elements are destroyed, after the costovertebral joints are severed, and after the rib cage is cut.[26] These effects were most pronounced during application of lateral bending loads and axial rotation. However, in clinical practice it is not known if the type of injury can be identified by measuring intervertebral motion.

The observation that damage to the intervertebral disks results in increased intervertebral motion, similar to the increases caused by sectioning the costovertebral joints,[27] suggests that motion measurements alone may not help identify specific soft-tissue injuries in the thoracic spine. Increases in motion caused by ligament or disk sectioning are of similar magnitude to the variations in intervertebral motion that occur between individuals. Without preinjury measurements of motion in an individual, it may be hard to tell if postinjury motions are abnormal or are within normal limits. Nevertheless, measurements of intervertebral motion abnormalities, combined with information about the type of loads that may have created the injury and the radiographic findings, can help clinicians differentiate between disk and posterior ligament damage. Clinical studies that assess motion at a segment relative to the amount of motion at adjacent segments may provide more useful data for assessing thoracolumbar injuries, although quantitative guidelines have yet to be developed.

Although data describing normal motion between vertebrae can be helpful in assessing potential problems, pain and/or muscle spasm may prevent a patient with a spinal injury from moving enough to create even normal intervertebral motion. Therefore, the lack of abnormal intervertebral motion cannot be used to rule out instability unless the gross motion of the patient is normal. Getting a patient with back pain to maintain a flexed or extended position during imaging studies can be very difficult. This problem has been described in clinical studies of patients with acute cervical spine injuries.[29] There are no accepted standards for imaging motion in the spine, so unless the physician directly supervises the imaging or has very high confidence in the technicians, the value of the intervertebral motion measurements may be limited. There are no accepted methods for measuring intervertebral motion during lateral bending or axial rotation. Even if a practical method existed to measure motion during lateral bending, axial rotation, or even axial loading, interpreting the motion could be complicated because of coupled motions in the thoracic spine.[24]

BIOMECHANICAL EFFECTS OF TREATMENT

The options for treating a thoracolumbar fracture can be broadly grouped into nonsurgical or surgical; these options are discussed in detail in other chapters. Nonsurgical options include observation, activity modifications, or external bracing. Surgical options range from relatively simple surgical decompression to extensive internal fixation with hardware to stabilize the spine and facilitate fusion. Each of these options can alter the mechanics of the spine.

Effects of Decompression

Surgery to remove fragments of bone that appear to compress neural elements may include laminectomy, facet resection, or disruption of the articulation between a rib head and the vertebra. Yoganandan and associates[30] reported in laboratory failure tests following a two-level laminectomy in cadaver spines that the laminectomy significantly reduced the load-bearing and energy-absorbing capacities of the spine, although the laminectomies did not significantly affect overall deformation of the spine. The authors suggest that the effect of a laminectomy would be more pronounced in the presence of a vertebral fracture. Similarly, Takeuchi and associates[27] reported that partial diskectomy can lead to large increases in motion between vertebrae, with motion increase seen in all three planes. Other investigators showed that resection of the facet joints, particularly the lateral aspects, results in increased intervertebral motion. Similarly, resecting a rib head resulted in even greater increases in intervertebral motion.[31] Biomechanically, a laminectomy alone is contraindicated for a burst fracture because the posterior column may be the only intact column. Similarly, the anterior column may be the only intact column after a flexion-distraction injury; therefore, surgical disruption of the anterior column is contraindicated.

Effects of Fusion

To prevent additional neurologic injury or deformity, fusion is considered the treatment of choice, with the ultimate goal of encouraging bone formation between vertebrae that will eventually be strong enough to prevent additional neurologic injury or deformity without the assistance of internal fixation or external bracing. To achieve this goal, internal fixation and/or external bracing is used initially to facilitate the natural adaptive capacity of bone to add to and remodel the fusion so that it is strong enough to provide the required mechanical support. To the extent that a successful fusion eliminates normal motion at certain levels, it also compromises the mechanical functions of the spine. Altered motion occurs adjacent to a fusion, especially at levels above the fusion.[32] However, the effect of this loss on the patient's quality of life generally is considered acceptable when permanent neurologic compromise or significant deformity is the alternative.

Several investigators have hypothesized that because of the potential need to compensate for lost motion, a fusion procedure may increase stresses at adjacent levels and thereby accelerate degeneration at these levels. In laboratory studies testing this hypothesis, several authors report that facet forces, intervertebral motion, and disk pressures are increased following a simulated fusion procedure.[33-35] The changes in forces and motion measured at adjacent levels following a fusion occur primarily at the level above the fusion[34] and increase with the number of levels fused.[33] Rohlmann and associates[36] found no evidence of increased mechanical stress on adjacent levels, and others have reported decreased motion at levels adjacent to a fusion.[32,37] Finally, accelerated degeneration has been seen adjacent to fusions in the cervical and lumbar spine.[38-40] The possibility that a fusion could result in symptoms many years later should be considered when assessing if fusion is the best treatment option and when deciding how many levels to fuse above and below the injury. The probabilities for adverse outcomes following fusion are not known, so a surgeon must now rely on subjective assessments of the risks and benefits.

Effects of Instrumented Fusion

The goal of instrumentation generally is to protect the fractured level and any intended fusion sites from excessive loads and motion until the fracture has healed and the fusion is solid. This can be difficult to achieve and requires careful planning. Instrumentation should almost always be considered in the context of load sharing where it supports a portion of the loads through the spine, with the mechanically intact or augmented parts of the spine supporting the rest of the loads. This load-sharing requirement for instrumentation systems is very important because most internal fixation systems cannot independently support all the loads applied to the spine for any significant length of time. In addition, completely protecting a region of the spine from loading inhibits the body's natural ability to restore load-bearing capacity to an injured musculoskeletal structure. This load-sharing requirement requires a mechanically competent interface between the implant and the vertebrae. Therefore, the two fundamental interacting considerations important to selecting an instrumentation system are the interface between the implant and the tissue and the ability of the implant to share the necessary amount of the loads long enough to facilitate healing.

Using cadaver models, several investigators have measured the overall stiffness of a motion segment or intervertebral motion following application of a wide range of fixation hardware.[41-47] The recommendation to instrument two levels above and below a fracture is commonly used. The biomechanical basis for this recommendation is that relatively large moment arms are provided when using instrumentation several levels above and below a fracture, and these moment arms allow the fixation to protect the fractured level from bending moments. Purcell and associates[41] supported a recommendation for hook-rod posterior instrumentation, and Kijima and associates[42] reported that use of a hook-rod system three levels above and below the injury provided the optimal fixation. However, there are many qualifications to this recommendation, with the most important being the rigidity of the fixation system, the quality of the bone adjacent to the fracture, how much load can be shared across the fractured level, and the mechanical demands that will be placed on the fixation.

Posterior systems are the most common type of fixation. Hook-rod systems have been studied extensively, although there are now many alternatives. The hook-rod systems rely on the posterior elements to provide the interface between bone and implant that shunts a portion of the load from the spine and through the rods. Thus, this type of fixation can only be directly applied to an injured level when the posterior elements are intact. Hook-rod systems provide minimal support to an injury unless the fixation includes several levels above and below the injury.[41]

These systems have been known to fail due to lamina fractures or pullout of the hooks. Failure can occur at loads well below the load-bearing capacity of the intact spine[43] and at a level that is within the physiologic range, so additional measures should be considered to help maintain applied loads below the load-bearing capacity of the construct. Segmentally wiring the rods to the vertebrae can significantly improve the stability provided by hook-rod systems.[44]

Pedicle screw fixation systems are now commonly available. In biomechanical laboratory tests, cross-links placed between rods have been shown to significantly improve the overall stiffness of the construct, particularly in lateral bending.[45] One potential complication of pedicle screw instrumentation is fracture of the pedicles during insertion of the screws. This problem is a much larger concern in the thoracic spine than in the lumbar spine because the thoracic pedicles are smaller and it is more difficult to insert the screws down the center of the pedicles. In a laboratory study, Kothe and associates[46] reported that fractured pedicles significantly compromised the ability of a pedicle screw construct to minimize motion at the site of a thoracic burst fracture. Posterior plate fixation of the thoracic spine is another option in some cases. Posterior plates attached with pedicle screws were shown to provide more resistance to lateral bending and torsion than hook-rod systems, although they were found to be inferior in flexion and extension.[47]

Summary and Conclusions

Although validated, definitive treatment guidelines have not emerged from biomechanical experiments and models, a substantial amount of valuable insight can be gained from the biomechanics literature. With support from this literature, the principles of biomechanics can be helpful in the diagnosis and treatment of thoracolumbar injuries.

Careful consideration of the type of trauma (load directions and magnitudes) that causes a thoracolumbar injury can aid in identifying the areas of specific damage and in selecting specific diagnostic tests. Imaging studies can identify possible structural damages and aid in assessing whether the spine is mechanically unstable. Estimations of the residual load-bearing capacity of the spine and the probability of additional neurologic injury or loss of alignment can be used to select an appropriate approach to treatment, surgery, or instrumentation that may be needed to optimize clinical outcome.

References

1. Wilcox RK, Boerger TO, Hall RM, Barton DC, Limb D, Dickson RA: Measurement of canal occlusion during the thoracolumbar burst fracture process. *J Biomech* 2002;35:381-384.
2. Kothari P, Freeman B, Grevitt M, Kerslake R: Injury to the spinal cord without radiological abnormality (SCIWORA) in adults. *J Bone Joint Surg Br* 2000;82:1034-1037.
3. Oner FC, Ramos LM, Simmermacher RK, et al: Classification of thoracic and lumbar spine fractures: Problems of reproducibility. A study of 53 patients using CT and MRI. *Eur Spine J* 2002;11:235-245.
4. Oner FC, van Gils AP, Dhert WJ, Verbout AJ: MRI findings of thoracolumbar spine fractures: A categorization based on MRI examinations of 100 fractures. *Skeletal Radiol* 1999;28:433-443.
5. Oner FC: vd Rijt RH, Ramos LM, Groen GJ, Dhert WJ, Verbout AJ: Correlation of MR images of disc injuries with anatomic sections in experimental thoracolumbar spine fractures. *Eur Spine J* 1999;8:194-198.
6. Heggeness MH, Doherty BJ: The trabecular anatomy of thoracolumbar vertebrae: Implications for burst fractures. *J Anat* 1997;191:309-312.
7. Panjabi MM, Oxland TR, Lin RM, McGowen TW: Thoracolumbar burst fracture: A biomechanical investigation of its multidirectional flexibility. *Spine* 1994;19:578-585.
8. Shirado O, Kaneda K, Tadano S, Ishikawa H, McAfee PC, Warden KE: Influence of disc degeneration on mechanism of thoracolumbar burst fractures. *Spine* 1992;17:286-292.
9. Fredrickson BE, Edwards WT, Rauschning W, Bayley JC, Yuan HA: Vertebral burst fractures: An experimental, morphologic, and radiographic study. *Spine* 1992;17:1012-1021.
10. Shirado O, Kaneda K, Tadano S, Ishikawa H, McAfee PC, Warden KE: Influence of disc degeneration on mechanism of thoracolumbar burst fractures. *Spine* 1992;17:286-292.

11. Albert TJ, Levine MJ, An HS, Cotler JM, Balderston RA: Concomitant noncontiguous thoracolumbar and sacral fractures. *Spine* 1993;18:1285-1291.

12. Kifune M, Panjabi MM, Arand M, Liu W: Fracture pattern and instability of thoracolumbar injuries. *Eur Spine J* 1995;4:98-103.

13. Wang JL, Panjabi MM, Kato Y, Nguyen C, Nguyen C: Radiography cannot examine disc injuries secondary to burst fracture: Quantitative discomanometry validation. *Spine* 2002;27:235-240.

14. Langrana NA, Harten RD, Lin DC, Reiter MF, Lee CK: Acute thoracolumbar burst fractures: A new view of loading mechanisms. *Spine* 2002;27:498-508.

15. Panjabi MM, Brand RA, White AA III: The three dimensional flexibility and stiffness properties of the thoracic spine. *J Biomech* 1976;9:185-192.

16. Hoshikawa T, Tanaka Y, Kokubun S, Lu WW, Luk KD, Leong JC: Flexion-distraction injuries in the thoracolumbar spine: An in vitro study of the relation between flexion angle and the motion axis of fracture. *J Spinal Disord Tech* 2002;15:139-143.

17. Hsu JM, Joseph T, Ellis AM: Thoracolumbar fracture in blunt trauma patients: Guidelines for diagnosis and imaging. *Injury* 2003;34:426-433.

18. Stagnara P, De Mauroy JC, Dran G, et al: Reciprocal angulation of vertebral bodies in a sagittal plane: Approach to references for the evaluation of kyphosis and lordosis. *Spine* 1982;7:335-342.

19. Korovessis PG, Stamatakis MV, Baikousis AG: Reciprocal angulation of vertebral bodies in the sagittal plane in an asymptomatic Greek population. *Spine* 1998;23:700-704.

20. Epstein NE, Epstein JA: Limbus lumbar vertebral fractures in 27 adolescents and adults. *Spine* 1991;16:962-966.

21. Mohanty SP, Venkatram N: Does neurological recovery in thoracolumbar and lumbar burst fractures depend on the extent of canal compromise? *Spinal Cord* 2002;40:295-299.

22. Gertzbein SD: *Classification of Thoracic and Lumbar Fractures*. Baltimore, MD, Williams & Wilkins, 1992.

23. Fontijne W, DeKlerk L, Braakman R: CT scan prediction of neurological deficit in thoracolumbar burst fractures. *J Bone Joint Surg Br* 1992;74:683-685.

24. Panjabi MM, Brand RA Jr, White AA III: Mechanical properties of the human thoracic spine as shown by three-dimensional load-displacement curves. *J Bone Joint Surg Am* 1976;58:642-652.

25. Panjabi MM, Krag MH, Dimnet JC, Walter SD, Brand RA: Thoracic spine centers of rotation in the sagittal plane. *J Orthop Res* 1984;1:387-394.

26. Oda I, Abumi K, Lu D, Shono Y, Kaneda K: Biomechanical role of the posterior elements, costovertebral joints, and rib cage in the stability of the thoracic spine. *Spine* 1996;21:1423-1429.

27. Takeuchi T, Abumi K, Shono Y, Oda I, Kaneda K: Biomechanical role of the intervertebral disc and costovertebral joint in stability of the thoracic spine: A canine model study. *Spine* 1999;24:1414-1420.

28. Panjabi MM, Hausfeld JN, White AA III: A biomechanical study of the ligamentous stability of the thoracic spine in man. *Acta Orthop Scand* 1981;52:315-326.

29. Insko EK, Gracias VH, Gupta R, Goettler CE, Gaieski DF, Dalinka MK: Utility of flexion and extension radiographs of the cervical spine in the acute evaluation of blunt trauma. *J Trauma* 2002;53:426-429.

30. Yoganandan N, Maiman DJ, Pintar FA, Bennett GJ, Larson SJ: Biomechanical effects of laminectomy on thoracic spine stability. *Neurosurgery* 1993;32:604-610.

31. Oda I, Abumi K, Cunningham BW, Kaneda K, McAfee PC: An in vitro human cadaveric study investigating the biomechanical properties of the thoracic spine. *Spine* 2002;27:E64-E70.

32. Lindsey RW, Dick W, Nunchuck S, Zach G: Residual intersegmental spinal mobility following limited pedicle fixation of thoracolumbar spine fractures with the fixateur interne. *Spine* 1993;18:474-478.

33. Nagata H, Schendel MJ, Transfeldt EE, Lewis JL: The effects of immobilization of long segments of the spine on the adjacent and distal facet force and lumbosacral motion. *Spine* 1993;18:2471-2479.

34. Bastian L, Lange U, Knop C, Tusch G, Blauth M: Evaluation of the mobility of adjacent segments after posterior thoracolumbar fixation: A biomechanical study. *Eur Spine J* 2001;10:295-300.

35. Eck JC, Humphreys SC, Hodges SD: Adjacent-segment degeneration after lumbar fusion: a review of clinical, biomechanical, and radiologic studies. *Am J Orthop* 1999;28:336-340.

36. Rohlmann A, Neller S, Bergmann G, Graichen F, Claes L, Wilke HJ: Effect of an internal fixator and a bone graft on intersegmental spinal motion and intradiscal pressure in the adjacent regions. *Eur Spine J* 2001;10:301-308.

37. Leferink VJ, Nijboer JM, Zimmerman KW, Veldhuis EF, tenVergert EM, tenVergert DH: Thoracolumbar spinal fractures: Segmental range of motion after dorsal spondylodesis in 82 patients. A prospective study. *Eur Spine J* 2002;11:2-7.

38. Hunter LY, Braunstein EM, Bailey RW: Radiographic changes following anterior cervical fusion. *Spine* 1980;5:399-401.

39. Lehmann TR, Spratt KF, Tozzi JE, et al: Long-term follow-up of lower lumbar fusion patients. *Spine* 1987;12:97-104.

40. Lee CK: Accelerated degeneration of the segment adjacent to a lumbar fusion. *Spine* 1988;13:375-377.

41. Purcell GA, Markolf KL, Dawson EG: Twelfth thoracic-first lumbar vertebral mechnical stability of fractures

after Harrington-rod instrumentation. *J Bone Joint Surg Am* 1981;63:71-78.

42. Kijima M, Sakou T, Nakanishi K: Dynamic analysis of the Harrington system using a spinal simulator. *Spine* 1990;15:1126-1130.

43. Maiman DJ, Sances A Jr, Larson SJ, et al: Comparison of the failure biomechanics of spinal fixation devices. *Neurosurgery* 1985;17:574-580.

44. McAfee PC, Werner FW, Glisson RR: A biomechanical analysis of spinal instrumentation systems in thoracolumbar fractures: Comparison of traditional Harrington distraction instrumentation with segmental spinal instrumentation. *Spine* 1985;10:204-217.

45. Lynn G, Mukherjee DP, Kruse RN, Sadasivan KK, Albright JA: Mechanical stability of thoracolumbar pedicle screw fixation: The effect of crosslinks. *Spine* 1997;22:1568-1572.

46. Kothe R, Panjabi MM, Liu W: Multidirectional instability of the thoracic spine due to iatrogenic pedicle injuries during transpedicular fixation: A biomechanical investigation. *Spine* 1997;22:1836-1842.

47. Rapoff AJ, O'Brien TJ, Zdeblick TA: Biomechanical comparison of plates and rods in the unstable thoracic spine. *J Spinal Disord* 1999;12:115-119.

CHAPTER 3

CLASSIFICATION OF THORACOLUMBAR FRACTURES

STANLEY D. GERTZBEIN, MD, FRCSC

As new imaging technologies have been developed, a better understanding of the pathology and mechanisms of injury of spinal fractures has evolved. Classifications have been based on morphology[1-6] or on mechanisms of injury.[1,7-10]

One of the primary concerns when evaluating fractures is determining instability. The degree of instability correlates with the severity of the trauma and places the injury along a spectrum. Instability may be defined as the inability of the spine under physiologic loading to limit displacement, which can cause both neurologic injury and pain. Failure to identify the degree of instability has both early and late consequences. In the early stage of care, unidentified instability carries a risk of injury to the neural elements. Instability in the later stages can lead to kyphosis and may be associated with chronic pain and possible neurologic deficit.[5] Stability depends on the integrity of both the bone and the soft tissues, so classification systems must recognize both these components. The pattern of injury also contributes information, providing clues to the degree of violence involved in the trauma and the extent and severity of the injury. The ideal classification system is capable of identifying the mechanism, musculoskeletal components, and severity of the injury and, with this information, providing an accurate diagnosis from which appropriate treatment strategies with predictable outcomes can be derived.

THE DENIS CLASSIFICATION SYSTEM

The early classification schemes of Nicoll,[4] Watson-Jones,[6] and Holdsworth[8] offered an understanding of thoracolumbar fractures, providing background for the development of contemporary systems.

In 1983, Denis[11] introduced the three-column concept (Figure 1). Understanding the involvement of each column in a given injury helped determine stability, treatment recommendations, and prognosis for various fracture patterns. The Denis classification system is well known and includes four categories of injury (Figure 2). The first category includes compression injuries with loss of height of the vertebral bodies. These injuries are usually not associated with neurologic deficits. The second group of injuries is classified as seat belt injuries because of the mechanism of distraction associated with seat belts in motor vehicle accidents. The third category includes burst fractures of various types, including rotational burst injuries. The last category is fracture-dislocations, involving flexion/rotation injuries, dislocations, and shear injuries. The Denis classification includes 16 subgroups and provides useful information regarding the morphol-

FIGURE 1

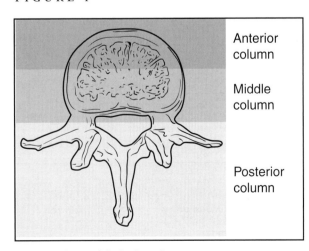

Anterior column

Middle column

Posterior column

The three columns of the lumbar spine.

FIGURE 2

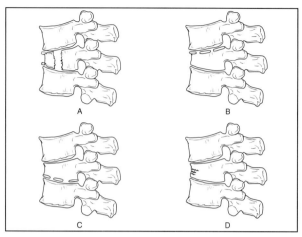

The four categories of the Denis classification. **A**, Compression fracture. **B**, Seat belt injury. **C**, Burst fracture. **D**, Fracture-dislocation. (Reprinted with permission from Garfin SR, Blair B, Eismont FJ, Abitbol JJ: Thoracic and upper lumbar spine injuries, in Browner BD, Jupiter JB, Levine AM, Trafton PG (eds): *Skeletal Trauma*, ed 2. Philadelphia, PA, WB Saunders, 1998, pp 947-1034.)

ogy and mechanisms of injury. Although this classification is used extensively, it has some shortcomings, as it is not organized according to a logical pattern of progressive instability, nor does it associate neurologic deficits with the various categories of injury.

THE LOAD-SHARING CLASSIFICATION SYSTEM

Based on a retrospective review of 28 patients with primarily burst fractures, McCormack and associates[3] developed a point system for assessing fracture stability. This system considers three features of the fracture—comminution, fracture fragment apposition, and degree of kyphotic deformity—and grades each on a scale from 1 to 3 depending on severity (Figure 3). Using hardware failure as the criterion, the authors found that segmental posterior instrumentation was successful in injury patterns totaling six or fewer points but failed in those that totaled more than six points. The authors suggested further stabilization in this group, either with a long posterior fusion or an anterior and posterior short segment procedure. Although the study has several shortcomings, it represents the only attempt to define the extent of skeletal damage that would predictably and favorably respond to isolated short segment posterior instrumentation.

THE COMPREHENSIVE CLASSIFICATION SYSTEM

First proposed in 1990, the comprehensive classification system is, as the name implies, the most comprehensive

TABLE 1

Comprehensive Classification of Thoracolumbar Fractures	
Type of Injury	Group
Type A—Vertebral body compression	1. Impaction fracture 2. Split fracture 3. Burst fracture
Type B—Anterior and posterior element injury from distraction	1. Posterior disruption, primarily ligamentous 2. Posterior disruption, including the arch 3. Anterior disruption
Type C—Anterior and posterior element injury with rotation	1. Vertebral body compression with rotation 2. Distraction with rotation 3. Rotational shear

FIGURE 3

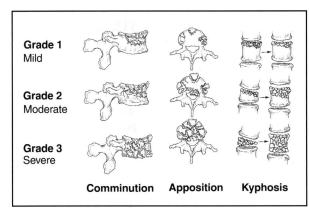

Load-sharing classification of McCormack and associates.[3] Fractures are assigned point values depending on the severity of three factors: comminution, apposition of fragments, and kyphosis. (Reproduced with permission from McCormack T, Karaikovic E, Gaines RW: Load sharing classification of spine fractures. *Spine* 1994;19:1741-1744.)

FIGURE 4

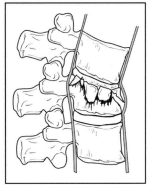
Type A

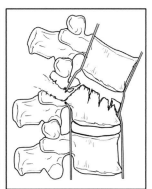
Type B

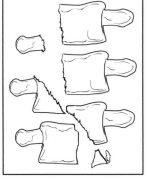
Type C

The three main categories in the comprehensive classification of spinal fractures. Type A, vertebral body compression; type B, anterior and posterior element injuries with distraction; type C, anterior and posterior element injuries with rotation.

system in current use[9,12] (Table 1). This system defines three basic types of injuries, types A, B, and C (Figure 4), each of which is subdivided into three groups.

Type A Injuries

Type A injuries are fractures of the vertebral body with compression, typically the result of an axial load with or without flexion. These injuries principally affect the vertebral body and are characterized by loss of vertebral height. Any fracture of the posterior elements that might be present will be a vertical split that does not substantially influence the instability of the injury. The posterior soft tissues are not disrupted, nor is there translation of the vertebral body.

Group A1 includes impaction injuries resulting from compression due to axial loading (Figure 5). This may cause an end plate infraction, a symmetric collapse of the vertebral body (osteoporotic fractures), or a wedge of the vertebral body superiorly, inferiorly, or laterally. Group A2 fractures (split fractures) occur with axial loading, resulting in a splitting of the vertebral body in the sagittal or coronal plane (Figure 6). The nucleus pulposus is forced into the vertebral body, causing the fracture to split, usually anteriorly. Because of the nucleus pulposus lying within the bone, a nonunion may occur. With group A1 injuries, the posterior wall is undisturbed, so neurologic complications do not occur. More violent loading may cause group A3 injuries, or burst fractures (Figure 7). Either one half or all of the

FIGURE 5

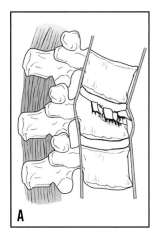
A

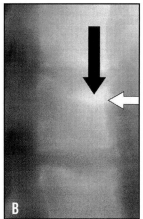
B

Comprehensive classification group A1 injury: impaction fracture. Diagram **(A)** and lateral radiograph **(B)** showing a typical wedge compression injury (white arrow) involving the anterior column secondary to axial compression (black arrow).

FIGURE 6

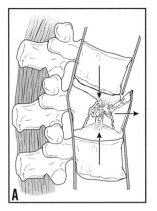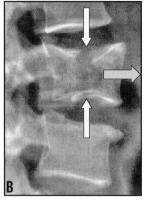

Comprehensive classification group A2 injury: coronal split fracture. Diagram (A) and lateral radiograph (B) of coronal split in the vertebral body that results in the intrusion of disk material from above and below into the substance of the vertebral body, forcing the anterior wall anteriorly and leaving the posterior wall intact.

FIGURE 8

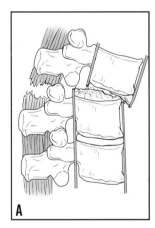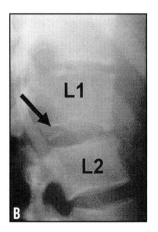

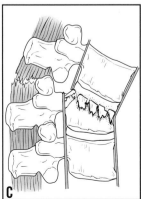

Comprehensive classification type B injury with predominantly ligamentous disruption posteriorly. **A,** Diagram showing how tensile forces result in disruption of the ligamentous structure posteriorly with propagation anteriorly through the disk space. **B,** On the lateral radiograph, the arrow indicates an avulsion of the posterior corner of the vertebral body as the line of disruption advances to and through the disk. **C,** Diagram of a similar injury associated with a vertebral body compression anteriorly.

FIGURE 7

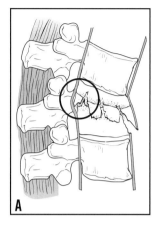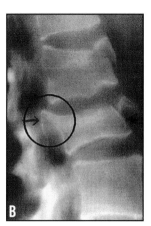

Comprehensive classification group A3 injury: burst fracture. Diagram (A) and lateral radiograph (B) showing an incomplete burst fracture involving the upper half of the vertebral body with fracture of the posterior wall and intrusion into the spinal canal by a posterosuperior fragment (circle, arrow).

vertebral body may be crushed, resulting in loss of vertebral height and often the extension of a bony fragment into the spinal canal with neurologic consequences. A vertical fracture of the posterior arch may occur, increasing the interpedicular distance. This latter injury does not usually increase the extent of instability. There is no rotation associated with any of the type A injuries.

Type B Injuries

Type B injuries involve all three columns, with the distance between the vertebrae being elongated by transverse disruption caused by distraction. Most of these injuries involve posterior distraction, but a small percentage are caused by extension and anterior distraction. If the axis of rotation is in front of the vertebral bodies, then distraction of both the posterior elements and the vertebral body will occur. If the axis of rotation occurs within the vertebral body, then axial loading will cause an anterior and/or middle column injury comparable to type A fractures along with posterior distraction. As can be seen, this classification system defines a logical progression of injury, with types B (and C) paralleling the type A pattern but with a different mechanism of injury and involving injury of increasing severity. Some injuries include significant soft-tissue involvement, which results in separation of the bony elements with increased interspinous distance or perched or dislocated facets. Translation may be present

FIGURE 9

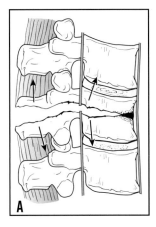 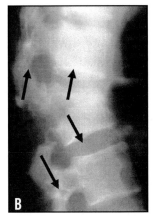

Comprehensive classification type B injury. Diagram **(A)** and lateral radiograph **(B)** showing distraction forces (arrows). There is failure of the vertebral body in tension and propagation of the fracture through the vertebral body.

FIGURE 10

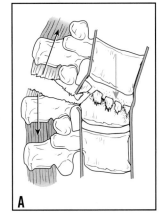 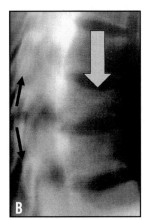

Comprehensive classification type B injury. Diagram **(A)** and lateral radiograph **(B)** showing the involvement of the bony arch (black arrows), associated with a vertebral bony compression anteriorly (gray arrows), similar to a type A compression injury.

FIGURE 11

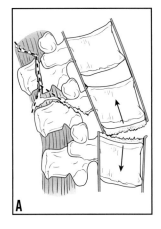 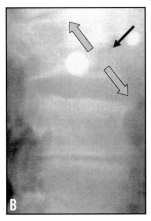

Comprehensive classification type B injury with anterior disruption. **A,** Diagram showing extension forces causing failure in the tension anteriorly, resulting in distraction of the spinal components anteriorly, predominantly through the disk (black arrows). This mechanism is associated with posterior disruption of either the soft tissues or the bony elements of the posterior arch. **B,** Lateral radiograph demonstrating anterior disruption with extension (gray arrows), causing an anterior inferior avulsion fracture of L2 (black arrow).

FIGURE 12

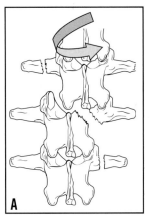 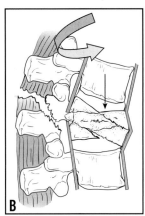

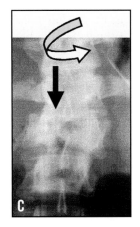

Comprehensive classification type C injury. AP **(A)** and lateral **(B)** diagrams and AP radiograph **(C)** showing the primary disruption force in this type of injury is torsion (curved arrows), which may be associated with axial loads (black arrows), as in this rotational burst fracture.

FIGURE 13

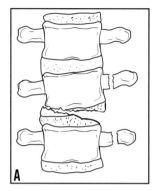

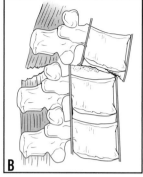

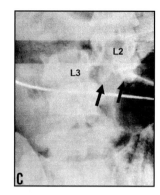

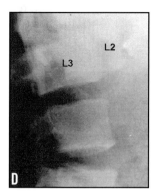

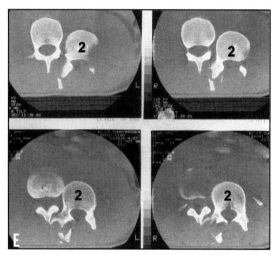

Comprehensive classification type C injury. The injuries illustrated here show that torsion may also be associated with distraction forces, as seen in any of the type B injuries. AP **(A)** and lateral **(B)** diagrams and corresponding AP **(C)** and lateral **(D)** radiographs show distraction with rotational force. Note that the facets of L2 are intact (arrows), indicating that distraction occurred before rotation. **E**, CT scans of the same injury demonstrate two vertebral bodies in the same place.

but only in the sagittal plane, and this is typically seen with dislocations.

Group B1 injuries involve a transverse posterior disruption of the soft tissues, and the injury may be propagated anteriorly through the disk, resulting in a subluxation or dislocation (Figure 8). If the transverse disruption through the posterior elements extends transversely through the vertebral body, the injury will be a variant referred to incorrectly as a Chance fracture[13,14] (Figure 9). In some cases, because of the axis of rotation being located at the posterior aspect of the vertebral body instead of anterior to the vertebral body, a type A pattern may also be present (Figure 10). A type B fracture is much more unstable than a type A fracture, however, because of the associated soft-tissue or bony injuries posteriorly, so it is particularly important to differentiate between type A and type B injuries. Although they have several common radiographic features, type B injuries are associated

with a much higher risk for posttraumatic kyphosis if not appropriately stabilized. Group B2 injuries are comparable to group B1 injuries except that the transverse posterior injury is through the bony elements rather than the soft tissues.

In group B3 injuries, the propagation of trauma begins anteriorly and is associated with hyperextension (Figure 11). Although more commonly seen in the cervical spine, this mechanism also occurs at the thoracolumbar level.

Type C Injuries

Type C injuries are associated with the most significant instability. In these injuries, both the posterior and anterior elements are disrupted by rotational forces. Like type B injuries, type C injuries are also three-column disruptions; unlike type B, however, they result in loss of instability in not just the sagittal plane but also the vertical and axial planes. In general, type C injuries include the injury patterns of types A and B, but the rotational component is added. Fractures of the transverse processes, dislocations of the heads of the ribs, and offset of the vertebral bodies and spinous processes are the key features of type C injuries (Figure 12). A fracture of the corner of the vertebral body may also reflect a rotational component. An oblique shearing mechanism may also occur.

Groups C1 and C2 include rotational compression fractures and rotational distraction injuries, respectively (Figure 13). Group C3 fractures are associated with rotational and oblique shearing forces (Figure 14), and these injuries are frequently associated with neurologic involvement.[15]

Advantages of the Comprehensive Classification System

This comprehensive classification system clearly defines fracture patterns and orders them according to increasing instability. Because the system takes into account soft-tissue injuries, it can predict the healing potential of the fractures. The classification also accurately reflects the relationship between the likelihood of neurologic deficit and increasingly unstable injuries (Figure 4 and Table 1): Although patients with type A injuries comprise approximately two thirds of thoracolumbar injuries, they represent only 14% of patients with an associated neurologic deficit; patients with type B injuries comprise 15% of the total fractures but represent 32% of patients with a neurologic deficit; and patients with type C injuries comprise about 20% of all of the fractures within this classification but represent 55% of patients with an associated neurologic deficit.[11] One disadvantage of the comprehensive classification system is its breadth, which makes it difficult to remember. Also, a thorough familiarity with the classification is needed to avoid inaccurate diagnoses.

RADIOGRAPHIC EVALUATION

Several factors must be considered when evaluating radiographs of thoracolumbar injuries (Figure 15). First, the vertebral body should be assessed with particular reference to its height. If a fracture is identified, the posterior elements must be evaluated for additional injuries. If no injury is present, or if only a vertical split is found, the fracture is classified as type A. If there is a transverse disruption of the posterior elements with no sign of rotation, the injury is classified as type B. If

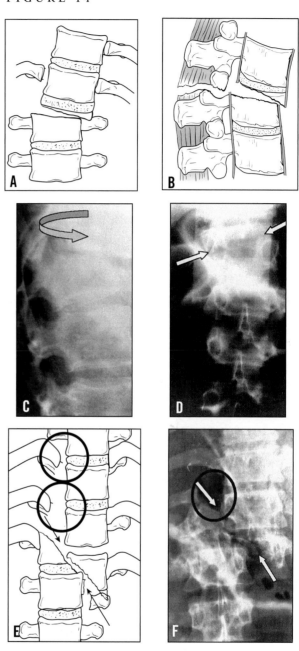

FIGURE 14

Comprehensive classification type C injury: rotational oblique fracture. AP **(A)** and lateral **(B)** diagrams and corresponding AP **(C)** and lateral **(D)** radiographs showing a rotational oblique fracture. This lesion is secondary to a torsional/shearing force resulting in a slice fracture (white arrows) as described by Holdsworth.[8] Diagram **(E)** and AP radiograph **(F)** showing a variant that is associated with a greater axial load than the slice fracture, resulting in a vertically oblique fracture of the body (arrows). Note the dislocated ribs (circles), which are associated with torsion.

FIGURE 15

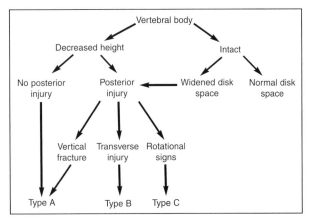

Algorithm for classifying spinal fractures according to the comprehensive classification system based on radiographic findings.

signs of rotation are present in the posterior elements, the fracture is a type C. If, however, no injury to the vertebral body is identified, attention should be directed toward the intervertebral disk. If a disruption is noted, the posterior elements must be scrutinized. Evidence of transverse disruption due to distraction injuries classifies it as a type B injury. If features of rotation are seen in the posterior elements, the injury is a type C.

SUMMARY AND CONCLUSIONS

Determining the instability of a spinal fracture is most important because the extent of instability dictates the method of management. Type A injuries, for the most part, are stable and do not usually require surgical intervention, with the exception of some burst fractures. Type B injuries, however, are more unstable, having the additional component of distraction along with flexion or extension and sometimes axial loading. These injuries require the principle of compression to restore their alignment and stability. The most unstable injuries are type C (rotational injuries), which usually require surgical intervention.

REFERENCES

1. Bohler L: *The Treatment of Fractures,* ed 4. Baltimore, MD, W Dood, 1935.
2. Kelly RP, Whitesides TE Jr: Treatment of lumbodorsal fracture-dislocations. *Ann Surg* 1968;167:705-717.
3. McCormack T, Karaikovic E, Gaines RW: The load sharing classification of spine fractures. *Spine* 1994;19:1741-1744.
4. Nicoll EZ: Fractures of the dorsolumbar spine. *J Bone Joint Surg Br* 1949;31:376-394.
5. Roy-Camille R, Saillant G, Sagnet P: Traumatologie du Rachis, in Detre T (ed): *Chirurgie, D'urgence.* Paris, France, Mason et Cie, 1976, pp 690-719.
6. Watson-Jones R: The results of postural reduction of fractures of the spine. *J Bone Joint Surg* 1938;20:567-586.
7. Ferguson RL, Allen BL Jr: Mechanistic classification of thoracolumbar spine fracture. *Clin Orthop* 1984;189:77-88.
8. Holdsworth F: Fractures, dislocations and fracture-dislocations of the spine. *J Bone Joint Surg Am* 1970;52:1534-1551.
9. Gertzbein SD, Court-Brown CM: Rationale for the management of flexion-distraction injuries of the thoracolumbar spine based on a new classification. *J Spinal Disord* 1989;2:176-183.
10. Whitesides TR Jr: Traumatic kyphosis of the thoracolumbar spine. *Clin Orthop* 1987;128:78-92.
11. Denis F: The three column spine and its significance in the classification of acute thoracolumbar spinal injuries. *Spine* 1983;8:817-831.
12. Gertzbein SD: Classification of thoracic and lumbar fractures, in Gertzbein SD (ed): *Fractures of the Thoracic and Lumbar Spine.* Baltimore, MD, Williams & Wilkins, 1992, pp 25-57.
13. Chance GQ: Note on a type of flexion fracture of the spine. *Br J Radiol* 1948;21:452-453.
14. Howland WJ, Curry JL, Buffington CB: Fulcrum fractures of the lumbar spine: Transverse fracture induced by an improperly placed seat belt. *JAMA* 1965;193:240-241.
15. Magerl F, Aebi M, Gertzbein SD, Harms J, Nazarian S: A comprehensive classification of thoracic and lumbar injuries. *Eur Spine J* 1994;3:184-201.

CHAPTER 4

SPINAL TRAUMA—INITIAL EVALUATION AND IMAGING

MITCHELL B. HARRIS, MD, FACS
CHARLES A. REITMAN, MD
PEDRO J. DÍAZ-MARCHÁN, MD

Advances in the treatment and transportation of trauma victims have improved the rates of survival; however, trauma remains one of the leading causes of death in people younger than 40 years. Trauma also continues to have a significant economic impact because it commonly affects those individuals with the greatest capacity for future productivity. Decisions regarding the early management of patients with spinal injuries rely on a complete understanding of the injuries, and imaging is an integral component of this initial evaluation. Although a detailed history and physical examination remain essential, advances in imaging have resulted in greater ease of acquisition and increased diagnostic accuracy, leading to new protocols for emergent evaluation of the spine. Appropriate imaging can facilitate decision making and expedite suitable treatment strategies.

EMERGENCY CARE OF THE TRAUMA PATIENT

The primary goal in the initial assessment of the trauma patient is to identify and treat any life-threatening injuries. To this end, the trauma ABCs (airway, breathing, and circulation) and protection of the cervical spine should be consistently observed. Airway control, enabling optimal oxygen delivery to the brain and central nervous system, must be established within minutes of the injury to avoid irreversible neural injury.

Second in importance, after gaining airway control and supporting the patient's ability to breathe, is the need to assess circulation. Aggressive fluid resuscitation is essential in the patient with multiple injuries. In the unconscious trauma victim, hypotension and bradycardia may be the first indication of a spinal cord injury (neurogenic shock). In this subset of trauma patients, oxygen, steroids, and vasopressors should be initiated after adequate initial fluid resuscitation has been achieved to minimize the insult to the central nervous system.

INCIDENCE OF SPINAL INJURY

Spinal column injuries are common among patients with multiple injuries. All patients with multiple injuries should be assumed to have sustained a spinal column injury and be treated accordingly until such injury is definitively ruled out. Approximately half of all patients with thoracolumbar fractures have associated multiple-system trauma. Nearly one third sustain injuries to one organ system in addition to the spinal column; 10% to 20% sustain injuries to two other systems; and 5% sustain injuries to three or more other systems.[1] Because of the urgent nature of an initial trauma assessment both in the field and upon arrival in the emergency department, these patients may have spinal column injuries that have gone unrecognized. In a retrospective review of occult injuries in the multiple-trauma population, Anderson and associates[2] found that thoracolumbar injuries were missed in 24% of their study cohort. Spinal injuries are more likely to be overlooked when the trauma victim is unable to provide assistance in localizing pain or is in extremis. Associated distracting injuries, an associated head injury, or intoxication with alcohol or street drugs at the time of presentation may also contribute to spinal injuries being missed.

Injuries to the thoracolumbar junction, which more commonly affect a younger segment of the general population, are the most common injuries to the spinal column. Mechanisms of injury include motor vehicle collisions, industrial accidents, falls from heights, gunshots, and sports. An estimated 15,000 major thoracolumbar injuries occur annually in the United States, with nearly one third resulting in an associated neurologic injury.[3,4] This anatomic area is particularly vulnerable because it is where the transition from the rigid, kyphotic thoracic spine to the mobile, lordotic lumbar spine occurs. The absence of ribs and the change in the facet orientation further predispose this area to mechanical injury.

EVALUATION OF THE SPINE

The comprehensive physical examination of the trauma victim includes a thorough evaluation of the spine. The goal of this spinal assessment is to identify and provide safe and expeditious management of spinal fractures that are potentially neurologically and mechanically unstable. The identification and management of spinal injuries is clearly secondary in importance to the trauma ABCs, but it should not be taken lightly. To accurately assess the spinal column in a trauma patient, a thorough physical examination, with emphasis on direct palpation of the spine and a comprehensive neurologic examination, must be combined with the appropriate radiographic studies.

Direct Examination

The clinical evaluation of the spine should follow a consistent pattern. Each portion of the spine should be palpated directly as well as inspected visually. This will require temporary removal of the cervical collar. All trauma victims should be logrolled to allow direct assessment of the condition of the spine by palpation.[5] Inspection of the soft tissue over the spine can often point to a specific area that requires more in-depth evaluation. Swelling, bogginess, malalignment, bony crepitus, bruising, and tenderness are all clinical signs of potentially unstable spinal injuries. Additionally, soft-tissue injuries on other areas

of the body can suggest a mechanism of injury that affects the spine as well. For example, the presence of a band of ecchymosis across the abdomen where a lap belt would be should alert the clinician to the possibility of a seat belt or Chance fracture. These injuries are commonly associated with acute local tenderness if not palpable defects in the posterior ligamentous complex that can be appreciated on physical examination. Throughout the palpation of the spine, the patient should be queried about the degree of local tenderness. Any report of tenderness should be noted, even in the presence of distracting injuries or in patients under the influence of alcohol or other recreational drugs.[6]

Neurologic Evaluation

A careful and thorough neurologic examination is essential in the trauma patient who is alert and cooperative. Accurate documentation of the patient's awareness of pain and ability to actively demonstrate motor function in a nerve root–based examination is a necessary component of the initial evaluation in the emergency department. A cursory examination that documents only the patient's ability to wiggle the toes is inadequate except in the setting of multiple injuries to the long bones of the lower extremities. Motor, sensory, and reflex testing results should be recorded serially in patients with suspected spinal cord injury or those who will require a lengthy initial surgical stabilization of injuries. Perianal sensation, rectal tone, and the bulbocavernosus reflex should be evaluated in all trauma victims, particularly those with a higher suspicion of a spinal injury. If a neurologic deficit is identified, focused diagnostic studies can be ordered.

Neurologic function is difficult to assess in the unconscious, intoxicated, or pharmacologically restrained patient. Spontaneous extremity motion and elevation of the rib cage with spontaneous respirations should be observed, as they indicate different levels of spinal cord function. Similarly, the patient who is unconscious or has altered mental status will respond to noxious stimuli with voluntary motor function (ie, withdrawal). Reflex arcs should remain intact regardless of the level of intoxication. However, spinal shock, defined as spinal cord/nervous tissue dysfunction due to physiologic rather than structural disruption, will eliminate these simple sensory-motor pathways below the area of injury; therefore, the potential for neurologic recovery cannot be predicted when spinal shock is present. Spinal shock can be detected by attempting to elicit the bulbocavernosus reflex by stimulating the glans penis or clitoris and assessing for involuntary internal anal sphincter contraction. Most commonly, the external stimulus is provided by gently pulling on the in-dwelling catheter. Spinal shock is generally considered to have ended when the bulbocavernosus reflex returns, usually within 48 hours. An isolated conus medullaris injury or mixed conus/cauda equina syndrome may directly injure the nerves responsible for the bulbocavernosus reflex, mimicking the presence of spinal shock. In this less common clinical scenario, the reflex may never return. In these patients, serial examinations and radiologic assessments are indicated.

Imaging

Spinal precautions are maintained until injury is excluded by reliable examination, which can include physical examination and/or imaging studies. Although algorithms for clearing the cervical spine have been investigated in considerable detail, similar guidelines do not currently exist for the thoracolumbar spine, and most protocols mirror the approach to the cervical spine. The patient who is alert and has no other distracting injuries and a normal mental status can be cleared on the basis of a completely normal physical examination combined with the absence of thoracolumbar pain. If the examination is abnormal or the patient reports symptoms, initial imaging is undertaken in the form of radiographs and/or CT. If no neurologic findings, midline tenderness, or significant midline findings on palpation are present and the patient is alert and cooperative, a normal radiograph or CT scan is sufficient to clear the spine. In the presence of abnormal midline palpation or neurologic findings, MRI is also necessary to clear the spine if the CT scan is normal. Any patient with a high-energy injury, which should be suspected with motor vehicle collisions in excess of 35 mph; falls greater than 10 feet; other fatalities at the scene of the injury; or injuries to multiple organ systems or multiple fractures, particularly the pelvis or the long bones, requires baseline imaging regardless of symptoms. There is a trend toward obtaining screening CT scans rather than traditional radiographs in this group of patients.

Patients who are obtunded are the most difficult to clear. This is controversial, and no specific guidelines exist for clearing the thoracolumbar spine in this population. Some physicians believe that the spine should never be cleared until the patient can cooperate with a physical examination. CT can exclude fractures with a high degree of certainty. Additionally, careful evaluation can often reveal alignment abnormalities that in the absence of a fracture would imply the presence of a ligamentous injury. MRI can more reliably rule out ligamentous injury but is often not practical or possible in the obtunded patient with multiple injuries. The same is true for weight-bearing radiographs. Decisions to clear the spine in this group of patients are usually based on the mechanism of injury, physical examination, and CT.

With rare exception, initial screening and evaluation of the spine begins with obtaining radiographs. Historically, the accepted standard has been to evaluate all trauma patients with orthogonal (AP and lateral) views of the entire spine. This is considered even more important in the trauma patient with at least one identified spinal column injury.[7,8] Depending on the patient's history, physical examination, and initial radiographic findings, advanced imaging studies may be considered. Findings on plain radiographs are sometimes obvious (Figure 1), but in cases where they are subtle (Figure 2), CT can frequently provide important information.

FIGURE 1

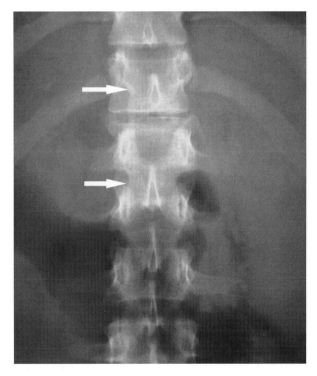

AP radiograph of the thoracolumbar spine of a 38-year-old woman who sustained a flexion-distraction injury when a patio roof collapsed on her. Note the interspinous widening between T12 and L1 (arrows). The patient was neurologically intact.

FIGURE 2

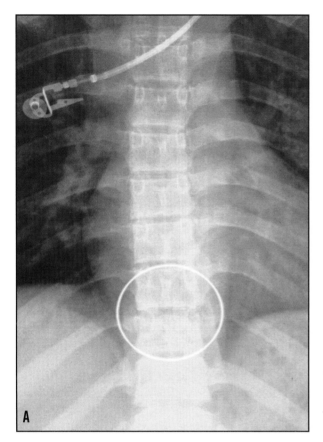 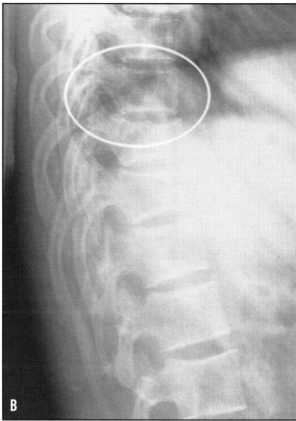

AP **(A)** and lateral **(B)** radiographs of the thoracolumbar spine of a 19-year-old man who fell 15 to 20 feet off scaffolding, landing first on his feet and then onto his buttocks. The only presenting symptom was severe back pain. On physical examination, acute midline tenderness was elicited. Radiographic findings are consistent with compression fractures at T10 and possibly T11. The patient also had fractures through the posterior elements and posterior ligamentous disruption, which are not evident on these radiographs.

Computed Tomography

CT has become invaluable in the assessment of spinal trauma. It has no equal in detecting injuries to the bony skeleton. With the new multidetector CT scanners, clear images can be acquired quickly and safely, regardless of patient size or position. Thin cuts should be obtained, preferably less than 2 mm, and axial images should always be reformatted into sagittal and coronal reconstructions. With these images, the spine is easily assessed for fractures, fragment displacement, changes in alignment, and degree of osseous injury. In distraction injuries, subtle signs of posterior interspinous widening may be present, and fractures of the posterior elements will be in the horizontal plane (Figure 3). These fractures are rarely seen in the axial cuts because they occur in the same plane. Therefore, it is important to review the reconstructions as well. The so-called "naked facet sign" may be present, indicating facet dislocation (Figure 4). In compression injuries, there will be no interspinous widening, and any fractures of the posterior elements will be vertical (Figure 5). One of the most common fractures involves the transverse processes. Isolated fractures of the transverse process are not unstable, but they are usually painful, and because they usually result from significant energy transfer, they are often associated with abdominal injuries as well. These fractures can often be seen only on CT. Beware of transverse process fractures coupled with contiguous spinous process fractures. Unlike isolated transverse process

FIGURE 3

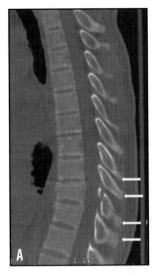
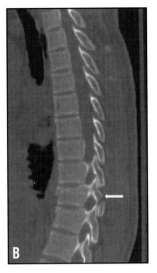

Sagittal CT reconstruction of the same patient in Figure 2. The axial cuts, which are not shown, indicated no posterior column abnormalities, a compression fracture at T10, and a very mild compression fracture at T11. However, the sagittal reconstructions clearly show the posterior fracture (arrow) **(A)** and subtle interspinous widening at T9-10 (arrows) **(B)**. Complete posterior ligamentous disruption was found intraoperatively. The middle column was intact, with compression anteriorly and distraction posteriorly. This was a flexion-distraction injury with the fulcrum centered at the middle column. The patient had no sternal or rib fractures.

fractures, these fracture patterns can arise from a rotational force that results in an unstable injury. CT nicely elucidates the degree of canal stenosis in the presence of a burst fracture (Figure 6). CT also reveals the complexity of some of the more unstable, rotational injuries (Figure 7).

Although CT is not the study of choice for evaluating disk herniations, it can be used when MRI cannot be obtained or is contraindicated. CT can also assess ligamentous injuries indirectly by revealing changes in structural relationships between adjacent vertebra. In addition, CT is the preferred study for assessing hardware placement and fracture reduction postoperatively. Indications for CT scanning are less well defined in the thoracolumbar spine than they are in the cervical spine. If a fracture is noted on plain radiographs, CT should be obtained to further evaluate and characterize the fracture. In addition, if thoracolumbar injury is suspected based on history or physical examination and radiographs are normal, the appropriate area should be evaluated by CT.

FIGURE 4

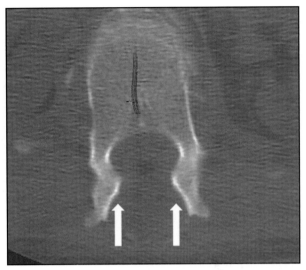

Axial CT scan of spine at T12-L1 level demonstrates a "naked facet sign," indicative of a posterior dislocation. At the L1 level, the inferior articular processes of T12 are not visualized.

Magnetic Resonance Imaging

MRI is unique in its ability to evaluate soft-tissue structures and is clearly superior to all other imaging in demonstrating ligamentous ruptures, disk injuries, hemorrhage, or spinal cord edema. It also provides good information regarding degree of stenosis (Figure 8). It is, however, generally less accessible, more time consuming, and less well tolerated by the patient than is CT. In addition, the presence of certain ferromagnetic devices precludes the use of MRI. Although it is used more often in the evaluation of the cervical spine, MRI can be very useful to help assess the degree of stability in the thoracolumbar spine by identifying ligamentous injury. This is important because determining the status of the posterior ligamentous complex is essential in the evaluation of the thoracolumbar spine, particularly when a distraction mechanism is suspected. MRI is also very useful in establishing the acuteness of osteoporotic fractures, particularly in patients with multiple fractures in different stages of healing.

The most common indications for MRI are in the assessment of neurologic deficits, particularly in patients with findings not clearly explained by CT, and to help evaluate degree of cord compression and injury. This will exclude the presence of an epidural hemorrhage, an associated disk herniation, or the rare spinal cord infarct. The presence of bogginess, a palpable step-off, or an obvious

FIGURE 5

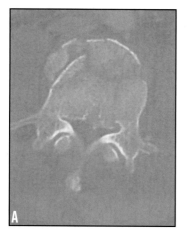
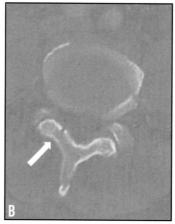

Axial CT scans of L3 of a 48-year-old man who fell 10 to 15 feet off a ladder while pruning trees, landing primarily on the buttocks. He reported moderate back pain but had minimal midline tenderness, and the neurologic examination was normal. The CT scans show a significant burst fracture (**A**) but no interspinous widening, along with a vertical laminar fracture characteristic of a compression injury (**B**). On the sagittal image (not shown), there was no interspinous widening. Despite significant canal compromise, the injury was stable and was treated uneventfully with bracing.

FIGURE 6

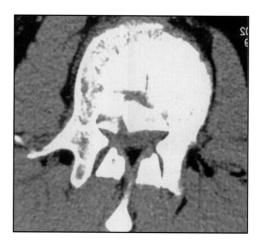

Axial CT scan of L2 of a 45-year-old man who was tossed around and buried by appliances when his trailer was struck by a tornado demonstrates a burst fracture. The patient reported severe back pain; the neurologic examination was normal. The patient was initially treated nonsurgically, with a thoracolumbar sacral orthosis. However, he continued to have severe pain that prevented mobility. Progression of collapse was also noted on weight-bearing radiographs. One week after the injury, the patient underwent a posterior-only short segment fusion. He was able to mobilize quickly after surgery. Although he ultimately had a residual kyphosis of about 10°, he was able to return to heavy labor 9 months later.

malalignment of the spinous processes on clinical examination suggests the need for further radiologic verification of the implied ligamentous injury.

MRI is also the test of choice in evaluating delayed, progressive neurologic deficits, and it can demonstrate chronic cord changes or cysts. Both T1- and T2-weighted axial and sagittal images should be obtained. Gradient echo T2-weighted sequences are preferred to the more traditional spin-echo sequences to evaluate for the presence of hemorrhage within the spinal cord.[9] In addition, a T2-weighted sequence with fat suppression nullifies the fat signal, thus emphasizing soft-tissue changes consistent with ligamentous disruption. If only limited sequences are obtained because of a "trauma MRI protocol," sagittal T2-weighted images are preferred because they generally provide more information than do the associated axial images.

Hemorrhagic findings on MRI change with time as the hemoglobin converts to methemoglobin.[10] Therefore, early MRI studies generally provide the clinician with the greatest amount of information. Axial MRI sequences allow direct evaluation of the spinal cord and conus medullaris and thus can provide early prognostic value.[11] Subacute MRI studies can provide the clinician with further information, including the extent of any spinal cord edema and/or hemorrhage, both of which are associated with poorer neurologic recovery.[12,13]

Flexion-Extension Radiographs

Motion radiographs are used as a means of evaluating instability in the cervical spine following trauma.[14] The same test can be performed in the thoracolumbar spine. Some researchers have studied stability in the thoracic and lumbar spines in the laboratory, but there are no proven clinical guidelines with established criteria for determining instability. In some institutions, flexion-extension radiographs are not used to evaluate the thoracolumbar spine. However, a similar concept is frequently used. In fracture patterns considered to have potential for nonsurgical management, radiographs are taken with the patient weight bearing in a brace and are compared with initial supine radiographs to assess stability of the fracture. Unfortunately, there are no specific guidelines defining degree of stability, but this strategy does provide information regarding the

FIGURE 7

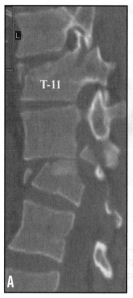
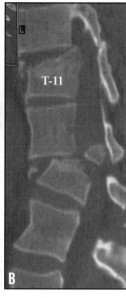
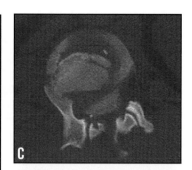
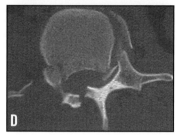

Sagittal CT reconstructions (**A** and **B**) of the thoracolumbar spine of a 42-year-old man who fell approximately 20 feet, sustaining devastating injuries to the spine and chest, resulting in a complete spinal cord injury with a level of about T11. Soft-tissue disruption was so significant that the pleura was discernible during the posterior exposure. Radiographs demonstrated a complex injury at T12-L1, consistent with a high-energy, type C injury (Gertzbein's classification). The CT scans (**C** and **D**) demonstrate the dislocation coupled with multiple fractures to all three columns. Also note the flexion-distraction injury at T10-11 that resulted in a fracture-dislocation.

tendency for the fracture and/or ligamentous injury to deform. Certainly the absence of motion or deformity is a compelling argument for continuing nonsurgical treatment.

IMAGING AND THE CLASSIFICATION OF THORACOLUMBAR FRACTURES

Imaging is integral to classifying fractures. Specific classification systems for thoracolumbar fractures are discussed in detail in chapter 3. One of the primary obligations of the surgeon is to identify fractures that have an element of distraction, which tends to make the injury more unstable. Because the injury is dynamic, the nature of the injury will not always be clear on static imaging. The posterior elements provide the most information in differentiating distraction from compression injuries.

SUMMARY AND CONCLUSIONS

A clear understanding of the biomechanics of the spine and proper characterization of the fracture are central to proper management decisions in the care of thoracolumbar fractures. Applying information from the physical examination and necessary imaging studies to this fundamental biome-

FIGURE 8

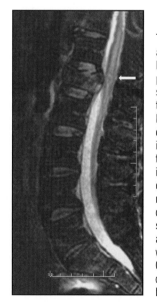

T2-weighted MRI scan of the spine of a 52-year-old man who fell off a horse, landing on his buttock. He had incomplete paraplegia on admission, with sacral sparing, weak but present rectal tone, and a motor level at L3. Increased signal intensity (arrow) indicates a burst fracture of L1 with an injury to the conus medullaris. Note the absence of posterior soft-tissue injury. The patient underwent anterior decompression and fusion only. He recovered bowel function but remained on a straight urinary catheterization schedule. He recovered anterior tibialis and gluteal strength but had residual weakness, 3/5, in the plantar flexors. One year after the injury, the patient could walk without assistive devices or braces.

chanical knowledge allows the treating surgeon to make an accurate assessment of the injury. CT in particular has become invaluable in providing comprehensive information and finalizing the evaluation process.

REFERENCES

1. Bauer RD, Errico TJ: Thoracolumbar spine injuries, in Errico TJ, Bauer RD, Waugh T (eds): *Spine Trauma*. Philadelphia, PA, JB Lippincott, 1991, pp 195-270.

2. Anderson S, Biros S, Reardon RF: Delayed diagnosis of thoracolumbar fractures in the multi-trauma patient. *Acad Emerg Med* 1996;3:832-839.

3. Benson DR, Keenen TL: Evaluation and treatment of trauma to the vertebral column. *Instr Course Lect* 1990;39:577-589.

4. Vaccaro AR, Jacoby SM: Thoracolumbar fractures and dislocations, in Fardon DF, Garfin SR (eds): *Orthopaedic Knowledge Update: Spine 2*. Rosemont, IL, American Academy of Orthopaedic Surgeons, 2002, pp 263-278.

5. McGuire RA, Neville S, Green B, Watts C: Spinal instability and the logrolling maneuver. *J Trauma* 1987;27:525-531.

6. Samuels LE, Kerstein MD: 'Routine' radiological evaluation of the thoracolumbar spine in blunt trauma patients: A reappraisal. *J Trauma* 1993;34:85-89.

7. Keenen TL, Anthony J, Benson DR: Non-contiguous spinal fractures. *J Trauma* 1990;30:489-491.

8. Calenoff L, Chessara JW, Rogers LF, Toerge J, Rosen JS: Multiple level spinal injuries: The importance of early recognition. *AJR Am J Roentgenol* 1978;130:665-669.

9. Sklar E, Ruiz A, Falcone S: Radiographic evaluation of spinal injuries, in Cotler JM, Simpson JM, An HS, Silveri CP (eds): *Surgery of Spinal Trauma*. Philadelphia, PA, Lippincott Williams & Wilkins, 2000, pp 127-150.

10. Hackney DB, Asato R, Joseph PM, et al: Hemorrhage and edema in acute spinal cord compression: Demonstration by MR imaging. *Radiology* 1986;161:387-390.

11. Bondurant FJ, Cotler HB, Kulkarni MV, McArdle CB, Harris JH Jr: Acute spinal cord injury: A study using physical examination and magnetic resonance imaging. *Spine* 1990;15:161-168.

12. Flanders AE, Spettell CM, Friedman DP, Marino RJ, Herbison GJ: The relationship between the functional abilities of patients with cervical spinal cord injury and the severity of damage revealed by MR imaging. *AJNR Am J Neuroradiol* 1999;20:926-934.

13. Silberstein M, Tress BM, Hennessy O: Prediction of neurologic outcome in acute spinal cord injury: The role of CT and MR. *AJNR Am J Neuroradiol* 1992;13:1597-1608.

14. Harris MB, Kronlage SC, Carboni PA, et al: Evaluation of the cervical spine in the polytrauma patient. *Spine* 2000;15:2884-2891.

MANAGEMENT OF SPINAL CORD INJURY

N I T I N N. B H A T I A, MD
F R A N K J. E I S M O N T, MD

Spinal cord injury has been a recognized medical entity for more than 4,000 years. The Edwin Smith Surgical Papyrus, dated approximately 1700 BC, includes case examples of vertebral fractures and dislocations with resultant paralysis.[1] This ancient manuscript describes spinal cord injury as a disorder in which the patient is "unaware of hands, penis is erect, and urine escaping unknowingly" and as "an ailment not to be treated."[2] Although many medical advances have been made since that time, spinal cord injuries continue to present treatment challenges and exact a significant toll on society.

Approximately 11,000 cases of spinal cord injury occur yearly in the United States.[3-6] At least one third of these patients will die either before or during hospitalization.[7-9] Recent advances, including the advent of model spinal cord injury centers, have improved the care of patients with spinal cord injuries during and after the acute hospitalization period. The average length of stay for patients entering a spinal cord injury center decreased from 26 days in 1974 to 16 days in 1999, and the length of stay in rehabilitation centers decreased from 115 days to 44 days.[6,10]

Spinal cord injury most commonly affects young adults, with the average patient age being 32.1 years. Additionally, most patients (81%) are men. Because of the young age of the affected patients and a postinjury employment rate of only 25%, spinal cord injury can have an enormous lifetime financial cost. Lifetime costs depend on the type of injury sustained, ranging from less than $500,000 for incomplete motor injuries to more than $2,000,000 for injuries resulting in high quadriplegia. The total cost for spinal cord injuries in the United States is estimated to be $4 billion annually.[11] The life expectancy for these patients continues to increase, but it remains shorter than that of the general population. Pulmonary complications are now the main cause of reduced life expectancy in this population.[6]

Data from the National Spinal Cord Injury Statistical Center[6] show that since 1973, the percentage of spinal cord injuries due to motor vehicle accidents and sports activities has steadily declined, whereas the percentage of injuries due to acts of violence has steadily increased. Since 1990, automobile accidents have been the most common cause of spinal cord injuries (38.5%), followed by acts of violence (24.5%), falls (21.8%), and sports (7.2%). At presentation, patients most commonly have incomplete tetraplegia (29.6%), followed closely by complete paraplegia (27.3%). The percentage of patients with complete tetraplegia (18.6%) is decreasing, while the percentage with incomplete paraplegia (20.6%) is increasing.

Spinal cord injuries associated with thoracolumbar fractures represent a specific subset of injuries. A thorough appreciation of the anatomy and fracture patterns of the thoracolumbar region, as well as knowledge of the pathophysiology of spinal cord injuries, is necessary to understand the management of these injuries.

ANATOMY

The thoracolumbar junction represents a transition point in the spine. The thoracic spine is relatively rigid because of the upper nine rib articulations as well as the coronal orientation of the facet joints. Because the 10th through 12th ribs do not articulate with the sternum anteriorly, however, there is less stability at the thoracolumbar junction. The long lever arm of the thoracic spine results in the increased forces that cause the various injuries seen at the thoracolumbar junction. In the cervical spine, it has been shown that patients whose vertebrae have small sagittal diameters are at increased risk for neurologic sequelae following trauma.[12] This relationship has not been found to be true in the thoracolumbar spine, although the overall shape of the spinal canal, as determined by the ratio of the sagittal diameter to the transverse diameter, may be predictive of spinal cord injury.[13] The relatively large spinal canal and rotationally resistant sagitally oriented facet joints in the thoracolumbar region help to reduce the rate of spinal cord injury.

The anatomy of the spinal cord in the thoracolumbar spine is unique as well. The spinal cord ends as the conus medullaris, which is usually located at the superior border of L1 in adult women and at the inferior border of L1 in adult men. The nuclei for the sacral nerves are contained within the conus, and their nerve rootlets as well as the rootlets of the lumbar levels continue distally in the spinal canal as the cauda equina. Injuries to the thoracolumbar junction can result in upper motor neuron lesions, lower motor neuron lesions, or combinations of both upper and lower motor neuron lesions, which is probably the most commonly encountered scenario. The clinical findings depend upon the extent of injury to the conus medullaris and cauda equina. Hence, a great variety of spinal cord injury syndromes can be seen at the thoracolumbar junction.

CLASSIFICATION

Thoracolumbar injuries can be classified by either fracture pattern or neurologic findings, as discussed in chapter 3. It is important to understand and differentiate among the various neurologic injury syndromes associated with these specific injuries.

Complete Spinal Cord Injuries

Complete spinal cord injuries involve complete paralysis and complete loss of sensation below the level of injury.

Acute spinal shock following trauma can mimic a complete spinal cord injury, but the conditions can be differentiated by the absence of the bulbocavernosus reflex in spinal shock. The return of the bulbocavernosus reflex, which usually occurs within 24 hours postinjury, signifies the end of spinal shock. At that point, the true neurologic status can be determined. Flaccid paralysis may occur, consistent with a lower motor neuron injury. If the spinal cord is injured just proximal to the conus, spastic paralysis and hyperreflexia can develop, indicating upper motor neuron injury. Complete spinal cord injuries carry a poor prognosis for improvement.

Incomplete Spinal Cord Injuries

Incomplete spinal cord injury syndromes are associated with partial motor or sensory loss below the level of injury. These injuries are further subdivided into central cord, anterior cord, posterior cord, and Brown-Séquard syndromes. Incomplete lesions generally have a better prognosis than do complete lesions with regard to neurologic and functional improvement.

Central cord syndrome occurs only in the cervical spine, but it is discussed here as part of the spectrum of incomplete spinal cord injuries. It occurs in patients with preexisting stenosis and disk disease. During hyperextension injuries, the spinal cord is compressed between the anterior osteophytes and the posterior ligamentum flavum. The centrally located spinal tracts are most affected, leading to greater weakness in the distal upper extremities than in the lower extremities. The overall prognosis for central cord syndrome is favorable, with most patients regaining both the ability to walk and bowel and bladder control.

Anterior cord syndrome involves the anterior two thirds of the spinal cord and results in paralysis and decreased sensation to light touch and pain distal to the level of injury. Sparing of the dorsal columns, however, allows vibration and deep pressure sense and proprioception to remain intact. Anterior compression of the spinal cord from displaced bone or disk fragments or from vascular insults can produce an anterior cord syndrome. This has the worst prognosis among the incomplete lesions.

Posterior cord syndrome is extremely rare and results from damage to the dorsal columns. This lesion results in loss of proprioception and deep pressure and vibratory sense. Motor function is retained.

Brown-Séquard syndrome involves a hemisection lesion of the spinal cord, frequently caused by penetrating trauma.

Motor function and proprioception ipsilateral to the injury are decreased, and pain and temperature sensation contralateral to the injury are affected. Brown-Séquard syndrome has the best prognosis of the incomplete syndromes, with almost 90% of patients regaining bowel and bladder function and the ability to walk.

Conus Medullaris and Cauda Equina Syndromes

The unique spinal cord and cauda equina anatomy encountered at the thoracolumbar junction leads to two additional types of injury patterns not seen in the cervical or thoracic spine: conus medullaris syndrome and cauda equina syndrome. Both of these syndromes present more discreetly than the complete and incomplete syndromes discussed previously. A thorough and complete history and physical examination, including rectal examination, bulbocavernosus reflex, and perianal sensation testing, is critical in all patients presenting with thoracolumbar trauma.

The conus medullaris represents the terminal portion of the spinal cord. Usually found at the level of L1 in adults, the conus contains the motor cell bodies for the sacral nerve roots. Injury at this level usually results in a lower motor neuron injury to the caudad sacral levels. Patients frequently have bilaterally symmetric perianal sensation loss. The loss of the lower sacral motor function also leads to decreased anal sphincter tone, absent bulbocavernosus reflex, and overflow bladder incontinence.[14] Lower extremity motor weakness is usually not a component of this syndrome. Prognosis is poor for recovery of bowel and bladder function.

Cauda equina syndrome can be caused by injuries in the thoracolumbar or lumbar regions. At this level, the thecal sac contains the lumbar and sacral nerve rootlets, from where they exit the spinal canal. Injuries in this region lead to sensory loss or radicular pain in a saddle-type or nerve root–type pattern. Motor weakness, flaccid paralysis, and loss of deep tendon reflexes also can occur, as can decreased anal sphincter tone, loss of the bulbocavernosus reflex, and overflow bladder incontinence. Because cell bodies are not affected in this syndrome, potential for recovery is much better than with the other spinal cord injury syndromes.

PATHOPHYSIOLOGY

Spinal cord injury involves both primary and secondary injury processes. The primary causes of spinal cord injury are the initial neural element deformation and energy transfer from the traumatic incident. Subsequent persistent neural compression may result in further primary damage to the spinal cord. Some injuries, such as missile injuries, result in only an immediate insult with no ongoing compression.[10]

The primary mechanisms of spinal cord injuries take place essentially immediately following injury and are due to the anatomic derangement and resultant vascular compromise, cell death, and axonal tract disruption.[15] A series of complex electrochemical shifts and ongoing localized blood flow changes lead to further acute cell death and toxicity. Immediately following the injury, significant decreases in blood flow occur at the site of injury,[16-21] although the precise mechanisms leading to this disruption are unclear.

The secondary mechanisms of spinal cord injury involve a complex biochemical cascade. These events are the subject of significant ongoing research. Various theories have been developed, each focusing on different causes of secondary damage, including systemic aberrations, free radical formation, calcium homeostasis, opiate receptors, lipid peroxidation, excitotoxic neurotransmitters, and inflammatory mediators. Most likely, secondary spinal cord injury is due to a complex interaction of most of these factors, as well as others yet to be discovered. Mediators represent possible targets for the medical treatment of spinal cord injuries. Because the secondary phase of the injury is a process that develops over several hours or days, successful intervention may be feasible.

The role of free radicals in these injuries has been studied extensively. Substantial evidence exists that oxygen radicals form after spinal cord injury.[22,23] These oxygen radicals ultimately cause cell membrane lipid peroxidation, cell membrane dysfunction, and cell death. Additional lipid peroxides and free radicals are produced by membrane lysis,[10,24] creating a positive feedback loop.

The accumulation of increased extracellular levels of excitotoxic neurotransmitters, including glutamate, as the result of both pre- and postsynaptic dysfunction, occurs soon after spinal cord injury. Prolonged glutamate receptor activation leads to an increased influx of calcium. Initially, this increased intracellular calcium is buffered, but eventually a rapid rise in the intracellular free calcium concentration occurs. The increased calcium causes enzymatic activation, changes in gene expression, cell membrane failure, and cell death.

Spinal cord injury results from a complex interaction of anatomic derangements and biochemical aberrations. Both immediate and delayed causes of spinal cord injury

FIGURE 1

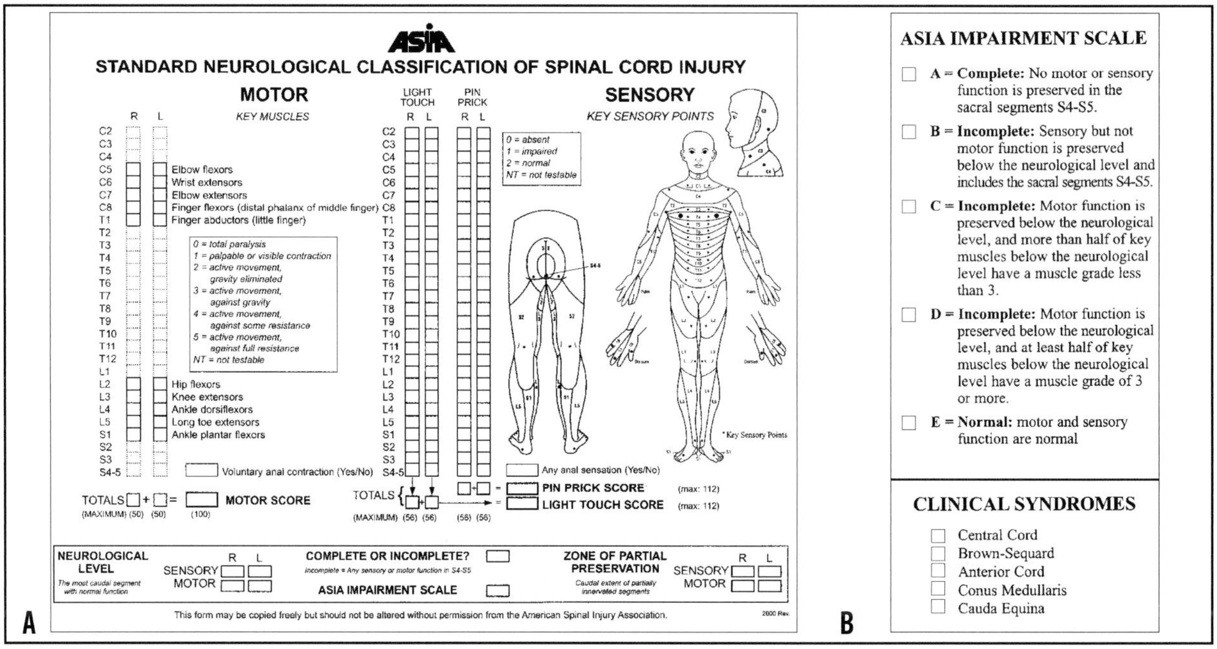

The American Spinal Injury Association's Standard Neurological Classification of Spinal Cord Injury Form. **A**, The first page of the form evaluates motor and sensory function as well as the level of injury. **B**, The second page classifies the level of impairment and clinical syndrome. (Reproduced from the American Spinal Injury Association and Research Foundation of the State University of New York, 2000.)

have been discovered, although the specific interactions and mechanisms remain elusive.

EVALUATION AND DIAGNOSIS

The evaluation and stabilization of patients sustaining thoracolumbar trauma is discussed in chapter 4. Several points are reiterated here that relate to spinal cord injury in particular.

A complete neurologic examination must be performed. Only a thorough physical examination can classify the specific type of spinal cord injury, which provides valuable information regarding the prognosis for recovery. The level of injury and any distal sparing should be clearly documented. Urodynamic evaluation should be performed to rule out occult neurogenic urinary tract dysfunction, which occurs commonly with thoracolumbar trauma.[25] Serial examinations should be performed regularly to assess for changes in neurologic status. Additionally, the patient should be reexamined after any treatment intervention because of the risk of decompensation after intervention.[26] The use of standardized grad-

ing systems for spinal cord injury, such as the American Spinal Injury Association (ASIA) impairment scale[27] (Figure 1), allows reproducible and understandable assessments of impairment. If such grading methods are used consistently along with serial examinations, changes in a patient's condition can be quickly recognized.

Imaging evaluation plays an integral part in the assessment of the patient with a spinal cord injury. Radiographs of the entire spine must be obtained to discern noncontiguous spinal pathology. CT and MRI can be used to delineate fracture patterns, soft-tissue involvement, and spinal cord edema. Furthermore, imaging studies provide important information regarding the injuries frequently associated with thoracolumbar spinal cord injury, including intestinal[28] and aortic[29,30] injuries.

MEDICAL MANAGEMENT

After initial stabilization and immobilization of the spinal cord–injured patient, management focuses on medical and surgical intervention to prevent neurologic deterioration and possibly improve existing neurologic deficits.

The medical regimen can be directed at the systemic effects of injury or at the spinal cord itself to prevent secondary spinal cord injury. Systemically, the goal is to prevent exacerbation of the localized ischemia found at the site of the injury, which can be made worse by systemic impairment of oxygen delivery. Oxygen supplementation should be given to keep saturations as high as possible. Additionally, systemic hypotension must be controlled. Neurogenic shock should be differentiated from hypovolemic shock. The former presents with bradycardia and hypotension unresponsive to fluid boluses. Hypovolemic shock, however, is due to significant blood loss, such as that seen in patients with multiple injuries in addition to spinal cord injury, and presents with tachycardia and hypotension. Once the correct diagnosis is made, the patient's blood pressure must be controlled. To prevent pulmonary edema and other complications, aggressive fluid resuscitation should be avoided. Instead, vasopressors and atropine are used to counteract the otherwise unopposed vagal tone encountered in neurogenic shock.

The secondary mechanisms of spinal cord injury lead to further neurotoxicity and spinal cord damage. Much research has been committed to identifying agents that can halt the various mediators of secondary spinal cord injury. Some of these agents are corticosteroids, glutamate receptor antagonists, opiate antagonists, and calcium channel blockers. Of these agents, only one corticosteroid, methylprednisolone, has been shown to affect spinal cord injury, and its role remains controversial.[31-38]

National Acute Spinal Cord Injury Study

In the 1970s, animal studies on the use of steroids with spinal cord injury showed encouraging results.[39] Additionally, the successful use of glucocorticoids to treat closed head injury suggested a possible use in spinal cord injury as well. These successes led to the first National Acute Spinal Cord Injury Study (NASCIS), which was a prospective, randomized, double-blinded, multicenter study published in 1984.[31,32] In this study, patients were randomized to either low- or high-dose methylprednisolone treatment. Low-dose treatment consisted of a 100-mg bolus followed by 25 mg every 6 hours for 10 days. The high-dose group received a 1,000-mg bolus and 250 mg every 6 hours for 10 days. No improvement was noted in the patients treated with steroids, and the high-dose steroid group had higher rates of wound infection, sepsis, and death, although only the difference in wound infection rates was statistically significant.

NASCIS II

In 1990, NASCIS II[33] was performed to evaluate the efficacy of higher doses of steroids than those used in NASCIS I. Like the first study, NASCIS II was designed as a prospective, randomized, double-blinded, multicenter study. Patients received either a 30 mg/kg intravenous bolus of methylprednisolone followed by 5.4 mg/kg·h for 23 hours, a 5.4 mg/kg bolus of naloxone followed by 4.5 mg/kg·h for 23 hours, or placebo. The study groups showed no difference in neurologic recovery at 6-month and 1-year follow-up.[34] When the patients were stratified according to when they were treated, however, it was found that patients who received steroids within 8 hours of injury showed better neurologic recovery than those who received naloxone or placebo. Wound infection and pulmonary embolus rates were double in the group treated with steroids, although this difference was not statistically significant. Interestingly, patients treated with steroids more than 8 hours postinjury showed poorer recovery than did patients treated with placebo.

NASCIS II[34,36] was the first prospective, randomized, double-blinded study to suggest that a medical treatment, specifically steroids, could improve recovery following spinal cord injury. Because of this study, steroids are used widely for the treatment of acute spinal cord injury. NASCIS II has been criticized, however, for numerous aspects of data analysis and collection. No patients with penetrating trauma, including gunshot wounds, or life-threatening comorbidities were included in the study. The stratification of the study population into groups treated before or after 8 hours postinjury was done after the study was completed. The differences in recovery were only noted in these post hoc subgroups, which were not followed prospectively during the study.[38] Furthermore, the improved neurologic recovery seen with steroids did not result in any functional or clinically relevant improvement.

NASCIS III

NASCIS III was a prospective, randomized, double-blinded, multicenter study that used three treatment arms.[35,36] Because NASCIS II suggested that steroids improved neurologic recovery, all patients in NASCIS III received a 30 mg/kg intravenous bolus of methylprednisolone at the initiation of treatment. After the steroid bolus, patients received 5.4 mg/kg·h of methylprednisolone for 24 hours, 5.4 mg/kg·h of methylprednisolone for 48 hours, or 2.5 mg/kg of tirilazad every 6 hours for 48 hours. In patients treated within 3 hours of injury, neurologic function was the same among the groups. In patients treated between 3 and 8 hours after injury, the 48-hour methylprednisolone treatment resulted in statistically improved neurologic recovery versus the 24-hour methylprednisolone treatment. Patients in the 48-hour group had higher rates of severe pneumonia and severe sepsis, although these were considered statistically insignificant. The NASCIS III results are subject to many of the same criticisms that were directed at NASCIS II.

NASCIS-Based Recommendations

The results of NASCIS II and NASCIS III led the authors to recommend that patients with acute spinal cord injury should receive methylprednisolone for 24 hours if treatment is initiated within 3 hours of injury or for 48 hours if treatment is initiated 3 to 8 hours after injury. Patients with spinal cord injury who are seen more than 8 hours postinjury should receive no steroid treatment. The controversy surrounding these studies and the use of steroids in acute spinal cord injury, however, remains quite intense.

Further Studies

Several additional studies have examined the relationship between steroid treatment and recovery after spinal cord injury,[40-48] with almost all suggesting that steroids do not improve neurologic recovery.[41,43-47] Furthermore, significantly increased serious complication rates have been found in patients treated with methylprednisolone,[47] especially when given for a prolonged period as suggested by the NASCIS trials.[49] Recent critical reviews of the literature, including analysis of the data from NASCIS II and III, have also concluded that steroids likely do not improve neurologic recovery and that they have significantly increased rates of serious complications, including death.[38,50]

The growing controversy surrounding the use of steroids in spinal cord injury has led many practitioners, especially in countries other than the United States, to abandon the practice. In a survey of Canadian physicians, only 36% of respondents followed the treatment recommendations laid out by NASCIS III. Of the physicians who prescribed steroids, 35% cited fear of litigation as the primary reason, and only 17% believed that steroids actually do improve recovery after spinal cord injury.[51] Adherence to the protocols of NASCIS II and III has also been problematic. In a retrospective review of 196 patients admitted to a spinal cord injury center in Ireland, only 28 patients received steroid treatment.[52] Of those treated with steroids, only six received the dose and time course of methylprednisolone prescribed by the NASCIS trials. A study from the United Kingdom showed that only 25% of patients who were candidates for steroid therapy according to the NASCIS protocol received the appropriate methylprednisolone.[53] An additional 10% received the steroid, but not according to NASCIS protocol.

Conclusions Regarding Medical Management

Although methylprednisolone continues to be used widely for the treatment of spinal cord injury in the United States, the controversy surrounding this practice continues to grow. The lack of reproducibility of the NASCIS trials and the significant side effects of high-dose intravenous steroids have led many practitioners to question or even abandon methylprednisolone treatment. At this time, however, it remains the only pharmacologic agent that has shown efficacy in human trials, and therefore it continues to be an important part of the armamentarium of the physician who treats patients with spinal cord injuries. At our facility, all adult patients with nonpenetrating spinal cord injuries and no contraindications to treatment receive steroid therapy according to the NASCIS protocol. Other pharmacologic agents for the prevention of secondary mechanisms of spinal cord injury are currently being investigated. The development of new agents or further testing of the efficacy and safety of steroids may clarify the role of pharmaceuticals in acute spinal cord injury.

SURGICAL MANAGEMENT

Indications for Surgery

Because of a lack of prospective, randomized, controlled studies evaluating surgery in patients with spinal cord injuries, many aspects of surgical intervention remain controversial. In deciding whether surgery is indicated, the four most important aspects to consider are: (1) current neurologic status and whether it is changing, (2) the presence or absence of spinal stability, (3) the presence or absence of neural compression, and (4) other non–spine-related considerations such as age, patient size, and comorbidities. Radiographs, CT, and MRI should be ordered as described earlier to adequately assess the fracture type, the extent of neural compression, and the level of stability.

Neurologic Status, Spinal Instability, and Neural Compression

One of the few areas of agreement with regard to the management of spinal cord injuries is that patients with neural element compression who demonstrate neurologic deteri-

FIGURE 2

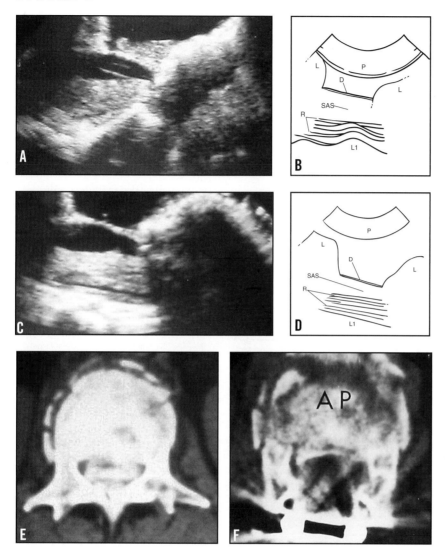

Ultrasonography and CT used to evaluate effectiveness of surgery for L1 burst fracture. **A**, Preoperative midsagittal ultrasound image of an L1 burst fracture with anterior impingement, and **B**, Diagram of the image. P = ultrasound probe tip; L = lamina; D = dura; SAS = subarachnoid space; R = nerve rootlets; L1 = L1 vertebral body. **C**, Midsagittal ultrasound image following posterior distraction instrumentation and posterolateral decompression shows the restoration of subarachnoid space anterior to the dura, **D**, Diagram of the image. P = ultrasound probe tip; L = lamina; D = dura; SAS = subarachnoid space; R = nerve rootlets; L1 = L1 vertebral body. **E**, Preoperative CT scan demonstrating the anterior compression on the thecal sac. **F**, Postoperative CT scan shows restoration of the canal and posterior instrumentation. (Adapted with permission from Eismont FJ, Green BA, Berkowitz BM, Montalvo BM, Quencer RM, Brown MJ: The role of intraoperative ultrasonography in the treatment of thoracic and lumbar spine fractures. Spine 1984;9:782-787.)

oration should be treated with emergent decompression and stabilization. In a patient with a neurologic deficit at the time of admission, enough neural compression, instability, or both is usually present to indicate that surgical treatment is appropriate. Patients with fracture-dislocations of the spine, with or without paralysis, will usually benefit from surgical reduction, instrumentation, and fusion. With rare exceptions, fracture-dislocations are very unstable and are best treated with posterior approaches. In general, the more unstable the injury, the more appropriate it is to perform posterior spinal instrumentation and fusion and the less appropriate it is to consider only anterior instrumentation

and fusion (Figure 2). Furthermore, the more unstable the injury, the more levels that will need to be included in the instrumentation and fusion.

Patients who have a burst fracture with severe neural compression, paralysis, and minimal posterior disruption are probably best treated with anterior decompression, instrumentation, and fusion (Figure 3). For these two extremes, injuries with instability as the major component and injuries with neural compression as the major component, a second operation on the opposite side of the spine could be performed if either the decompression, in the former case, or the stabilization, in the latter case, was not adequate (Figure 4).

FIGURE 3

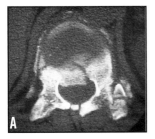
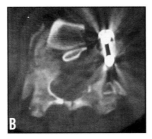

CT scan of a patient who sustained a T12 burst fracture with an incomplete neurologic injury after ejection from a military aircraft. Because of the significant canal compromise, neurologic injury, and burns involving a significant portion of the patient's back, anterior decompression and stabilization was performed. **A**, Preoperative CT scan demonstrates the T12 burst fracture with canal compromise. **B**, Postoperative CT scan shows decompression of the spinal canal along with anterior bone graft and instrumentation. The patient returned to flying approximately 1 year after the injury.

Other Patient Considerations

If the patient is obese or if the surgeon thinks that the instability is severe, the bone quality is poor, or the postoperative demands are great because of comorbidities, posterior surgery is even more appropriate. Extra levels of posterior instrumentation are likely to be indicated as well.

Spinal Angulation

Spinal angulation of more than 30° should always be treated surgically to prevent chronic back pain. Angulation of 25° to 30° may require surgical treatment, although this degree of deformity can be treated nonsurgically if the patient is followed closely and is informed that the angulation may progress and require surgical correction later.

Instrumentation Systems

Many systems are adequate for anterior instrumentation and fusion. In general, autogenous bone graft will heal more rapidly and predictably than allograft. For posterior instrumentation and fusion, pedicle screws and rods provide a more rigid construct and lose less correction over time than do hook constructs. For further discussion of instrumentation systems, see chapter 7.

Timing of Nonemergent Surgery

In patients with a stable neurologic deficit and neural compression, the appropriate timing of surgical inter-

FIGURE 4

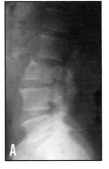
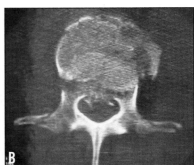
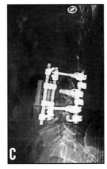
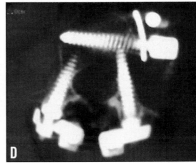

Imaging evaluation of a patient who sustained an L3 burst fracture with paraparesis after being struck by a car. The surgery was delayed because of alcohol withdrawal and delirium. **A**, Preoperative lateral radiograph reveals an L3 burst fracture with severe retrolisthesis, loss of L2 on L3 height, and kyphosis. **B**, Preoperative CT scan shows canal compromise and anterior comminution. **C**, Postoperative lateral radiograph following anterior decompression and anterior and posterior instrumentation. Note the restoration of height and lordosis in the lumbar spine and the improved alignment. Anterior and posterior instrumentation were used because of the marked anterior and posterior disruption and lack of dependability of the patient. **D**, Postoperative CT scan demonstrates the anterior and posterior instrumentation.

vention is controversial. Animal studies[54] have suggested that early decompression may improve neurologic recovery. These results, however, have not been replicated in humans. Numerous studies[55-59] have evaluated the effect of timing of decompression on neurologic recovery in humans, but these investigations have not provided conclusive evidence supporting either early or delayed decompression of patients with nondeteriorating spinal cord injuries. This lack of consensus has led to wide variations in the timing of surgical intervention for spinal cord injuries.[60] These patients frequently have significant comorbidities, and care must be taken to ensure that they are medically optimized before surgical intervention.[26,61]

Summary and Conclusions

Spinal cord injuries associated with thoracolumbar fractures continue to be a significant problem. Damage to the spinal cord likely occurs both from the trauma itself and from the secondary biochemical cascade caused by the injury. Detailed serial examinations, a complete imaging work-up, aggressive medical resuscitation, and immobilization of the spine are critical aspects in the care of the spinal cord–injured patient. Many aspects of the pharmacologic and surgical treatment of these patients remain controversial, but recent advances have significantly improved outcomes following these injuries.

References

1. Feldman RP, Goodrich JT: The Edwin Smith Surgical Papyrus. *Childs Nerv Syst* 1999;15:281-284.

2. Breasted JH: *The Edwin Smith Surgical Papyrus.* Chicago, IL, University of Chicago Press, 1930.

3. Kraus JF, Franti CE, Riggins RS, Richards D, Borhani NO: Incidence of traumatic spinal cord lesions. *J Chronic Dis* 1975;28:471-492.

4. Woolsey RM: Modern concepts of therapy and management of spinal cord injuries. *Crit Rev Neurobiol* 1988;4:137-156.

5. Ergas Z: Spinal cord injury in the United States: A statistical update. *Cent Nerv Syst Trauma* 1985;2:19-32.

6. National Spinal Cord Injury Statistical Center: Spinal Cord Injury: Facts and Figures at a Glance. Birmingham, Alabama, University of Alabama at Birmingham, 2001.

7. Albin MS, White RJ: Epidemiology, physiopathology, and experimental therapeutics of acute spinal cord injury. *Crit Care Clin* 1987;3:441-452.

8. Carter RE: Etiology of traumatic spinal cord injury: Statistics of more than 1,100 cases. *Tex Med* 1977;73:61-65.

9. Kraus JF: Epidemiologic features of head and spinal cord injury. *Adv Neurol* 1978;19:261-279.

10. Sekhon LH, Fehlings MG: Epidemiology, demographics, and pathophysiology of acute spinal cord injury. *Spine* 2001;26(suppl):2-12.

11. Stripling TE: The cost of economic consequences of traumatic spinal cord injury. *Paraplegia News* 1990;8:50-54.

12. Eismont FJ, Clifford S, Goldberg M, Green B: Cervical sagittal spinal canal size in spine injury. *Spine* 1984;9:663-666.

13. Vaccaro AR, Nachwalter RS, Klein GR, Sewards JM, Albert TJ, Garfin SR: The significance of thoracolumbar spinal canal size in spinal cord injury patients. *Spine* 2001;26:371-376.

14. Haher TR, Felmly WT, O'Brien M: Thoracic and lumbar fractures: Diagnosis and management, in Bridwell KH, Dewald RL, Hammerberg KW, et al (eds): *The Textbook of Spinal Surgery,* ed 2. New York, NY, Lippincott Williams & Wilkins, 1997, pp 1773-1778.

15. Delamarter RB, Coyle J: Acute management of spinal cord injury. *J Am Acad Orthop Surg* 1999;7:166-175.

16. Bingham WG, Goldman H, Friedman SJ, Murphy S, Yashon D, Hunt WE: Blood flow in the normal and injured monkey spinal cord. *J Neurosurg* 1975;43:162-171.

17. Griffiths IR: Spinal cord blood flow after acute experimental cord injury in dogs. *J Neurol Sci* 1976;27:247-259.

18. Kobrine AI, Koyle TF, Martins AN: Local spinal cord blood flow in experimental traumatic myelopathy. *J Neurosurg* 1975;42:144-149.

19. Senter HJ, Venes JL: Altered blood flow and secondary injury in experimental spinal cord trauma. *J Neurosurg* 1978;49:569-578.

20. Tator CH, Fehlings MG: Review of the secondary injury theory of acute spinal cord trauma with emphasis on vascular mechanisms. *J Neurosurg* 1991;75:15-26.

21. Atkinson PP, Atkinson JL: Spinal shock. *Mayo Clin Proc* 1996;71:384-389.

22. Demopoulos HB, Flamm ES, Pietronigro DD, Seligman ML: The free radical pathology and the microcirculation in the major central nervous system disorders. *Acta Physiol Scand Suppl* 1980;492:91-119.

23. Demopoulos HB, Flamm ES, Seligman ML, Pietronigro DD, Tomasula J, DeCrescito V: Further studies on free-radical pathology in the major central nervous system disorders: Effect of very high doses of methylprednisolone on the functional outcome, morphology, and chemistry of experimental spinal cord impact injury. *Can J Physiol Pharmacol* 1982;60:1415-1424.

24. Hall ED, Braughler JM: Free radicals in CNS injury. *Res Publ Assoc Res Nerv Ment Dis* 1993;71:81-105.

25. Watanabe T, Vaccaro A, Kumon H, Welch W, Rivas D, Chancellor M: High incidence of occult neurogenic bladder dysfunction in neurologically intact patients with thoracolumbar spinal injuries. *J Urol* 1998;159:965-968.

26. Marshall LF, Knowlton S, Garfin SR, et al: Deterioration following spinal cord injury: A multicenter study. *J Neurosurg* 1987;66:400-404.

27. American College of Surgeons: *Advanced Trauma Life Support,* ed 5. Chicago, IL, American College of Surgeons, 1995.

28. Anderson PA, Rivara FP, Maier RV, Drake C: The epidemiology of seatbelt-associated injuries. *J Trauma* 1991;31:60-67.

29. Ayella RJ, Hankins JR, Turney SZ, Cowley RA: Ruptured thoracic aorta due to blunt trauma. *J Trauma* 1977;17:199-205.

30. Mohinder PSR, Menzoian JO: Seat belt aorta. *Ann Vasc Surg* 1990;4:370-377.

31. Bracken MB, Collins WF, Freeman DF, et al: Efficacy of methylprednisolone in acute spinal cord injury. *JAMA* 1984;251:45-52.

32. Bracken MB, Shepard MJ, Hellenbrand KG, et al: Methylprednisolone and neurological function 1 year after spinal cord injury: Results of the National Acute Spinal Cord Injury Study. *J Neurosurg* 1985;63:704-713.

33. Bracken MB, Shepard MJ, Collins WF, et al: A randomized, controlled trial of methylprednisolone or naloxone in the treatment of acute spinal-cord injury: Results of the Second National Acute Spinal Cord Injury Study. *N Engl J Med* 1990;322:1405-1411.

34. Bracken MB, Shepard MJ, Collins WF Jr, et al: Methylprednisolone or naloxone treatment after acute spinal cord injury: 1-year follow-up data. Results of the second National Acute Spinal Cord Injury Study. *J Neurosurg* 1992;76:23-31.

35. Bracken MB, Shepard MJ, Holford TR, et al: Administration of methylprednisolone for 24 or 48 hours or tirilazad mesylate for 48 hours in the treatment of acute spinal cord injury: Results of the Third National Acute Spinal Cord Injury Randomized Controlled Trial. National Acute Spinal Cord Injury Study. *JAMA* 1997;277:1597-1604.

36. Bracken MB, Shepard MJ, Holford TR, et al: Administration of methylprednisolone for 24 or 48 hours or tirilazad mesylate for 48 hours in the treatment of acute spinal cord injury: Results of the Third National Acute Spinal Cord Injury Randomized Controlled Trial. National Acute Spinal Cord Injury Study. *J Neurosurg* 1998;89:699-706.

37. Hurlbert RJ: The role of steroids in acute spinal cord injury: An evidence-based analysis. *Spine* 2001;26(suppl):39-46.

38. Hurlbert RJ: Methylprednisolone for acute spinal cord injury: An inappropriate standard of care. *J Neurosurg* 2000;93:1-7.

39. Eidelberg E, Staten E, Watkins CJ, Smith JS: Treatment of experimental spinal cord injury in ferrets. *Surg Neurol* 1976;6:243-246.

40. Kiwerski JE: Application of dexamethasone in the treatment of acute spinal cord injury. *Injury* 1993;24:457-460.

41. George ER, Scholten DJ, Buechler CM, Jordan-Tibbs J, Mattice C, Albrecht RM: Failure of methylprednisolone to improve the outcome of spinal cord injuries. *Am Surg* 1995;61:659-664.

42. Otani K, Abe H, Kadoya S: Beneficial effect of methylprednisolone sodium succinate in the treatment of acute spinal cord injury. *Sekitsu Sekizui* 1994;7:633-647.

43. Prendergast MR, Saxe JM, Ledgerwood AM, Lucas CE, Lucas WF: Massive steroids do not reduce the zone of injury after penetrating spinal cord injury. *J Trauma* 1994;37:576-579.

44. Poynton AR, O'Farrell DA, Shannon F, Murray P, McManus F, Walsh MG: An evaluation of the factors affecting neurological recovery following spinal cord injury. *Injury* 1997;28:545-548.

45. Pointillart V, Petitjean ME, Wiart L, et al: Pharmacological therapy of spinal cord injury during the acute phase. *Spinal Cord* 2000;38:71-76.

46. Pollard ME, Apple DF: Factors associated with improved neurologic outcomes in patients with incomplete tetraplegia. *Spine* 2003;28:33-39.

47. Matsumoto T, Tamaki T, Kawakami M, Yoshida M, Ando M, Yamada H: Early complications of high-dose methylprednisolone sodium succinate treatment in the follow-up of acute cervical spinal cord injury. *Spine* 2001;26:426-430.

48. Zigler JE, Anderson PA, Boden SD, Bridwell KH, Vaccaro AR: What's new in spine surgery. *J Bone Joint Surg Am* 2003;85:1626-1636.

49. Molano Mdel R, Broton JG, Bean JA, Calancie B: Complications associated with the prophylactic use of methylprednisolone during surgical stabilization after spinal cord injury. *J Neurosurg* 2002;96:267-272.

50. Short DJ, El Masry WS, Jones PW: High dose methylprednisolone in the management of acute spinal cord injury: A systematic review from a clinical perspective. *Spinal Cord* 2000;38:273-286.

51. Hugenholtz H, Cass DE, Dvorak MF, et al: High-dose methylprednisolone for acute closed spinal cord injury: Only a treatment option. *Can J Neurol Sci* 2002;29:227-235.

52. O'Connor PA, McCormack O, Gavin C, et al: Methylprednisolone in acute spinal cord injuries. *Ir J Med Sci* 2003;172:24-26.

53. Molloy S, Middleton F, Casey AT: Failure to administer methylprednisolone for acute traumatic spinal cord injury: A prospective audit of 100 patients from a regional spinal injuries unit. *Injury* 2002;33:575-578.

54. Delamarter RB, Sherman J, Carr JB: Pathophysiology of spinal cord injury: Recovery after immediate and delayed compression. *J Bone Joint Surg Am* 1995;77:1042-1049.

55. Fehlings MG, Sekhon LH, Tator C: The role and timing of decompression in acute spinal cord injury: What do we know? What should we do? *Spine* 2001;26 (Suppl):101-110.

56. Hadley MN, Fitzpatrick BC, Sonntag VK, Browner CM: Facet fracture-dislocation injuries of the cervical spine. *Neurosurgery* 1992;30:661-666.

57. Aebi M, Mohler J, Zach GA, Morscher E: Indication, surgical technique, and results of 100 surgically-treated fractures and fracture-dislocations of the cervical spine. *Clin Orthop* 1986;203:244-257.

58. Bohlman HH, Freehafer A: Late anterior decompression of spinal cord injuries. *J Bone Joint Surg Am* 1979;57:1025.

59. Bohlman HH, Kirkpatrick JS, Delamarter RB, Leventhal M: Anterior decompression for late pain and paralysis after fractures of the thoracolumbar spine. *Clin Orthop* 1994;300:24-29.

60. Tator CH, Fehlings MG, Thorpe K, Taylor W: Current use and timing of spinal surgery for management of acute spinal surgery for management of acute spinal cord injury in North America: Results of a retrospective multi-center study. *J Neurosurg* 1999;91 (Suppl):12-18.

61. Wilmot CB, Hall KM: Evaluation of the acute management of tetraplegia: Conservative versus surgical treatment. *Paraplegia* 1986;24:148-153.

CHAPTER 6

NONSURGICAL TREATMENT OF THORACOLUMBAR FRACTURES

CHRISTOPHER M. BONO, MD
JAMES ROBERT ALBERTS, MD
STEVEN R. GARFIN, MD

The earliest treatments of thoracolumbar fractures were nonsurgical, specifically, manipulative closed reduction, extended periods of recumbency, and plaster of Paris body casts. Many of these techniques have become obsolete; others have evolved into modern methods of nonsurgical fracture management such as custom-molded plastic shell orthoses. In recent years, surgical management of spinal fractures has gained substantial popularity, driven at least in part by the availability and versatility of thoracolumbar instrumentation. Thus, the purported indications for surgical treatment seem to be expanding, whereas interest and understanding of nonsurgical fracture care is dwindling.

Despite this trend, it remains true that most thoracolumbar fractures can be treated nonsurgically. Treatment decisions require information obtained from a careful physical examination and appropriate imaging studies. Guided by an understanding of the admittedly somewhat vague and variable biomechanical principles of fracture stability, an examination of the literature regarding these fractures can help define an effective nonsurgical treatment plan.

PATIENT EVALUATION

History and Physical Examination

The first steps in treatment planning are a careful history and physical examination. The mechanism of injury may be discerned from information about the type and direction of impact or injury. For example, in motor vehicle accidents, seat-belted passengers would be expected to have a more focal concentration of forces in the lumbar spine than would unrestrained passengers. Individuals who fall from a horse or over motorcycle handlebars may have injuries at the thoracolumbar junction. Although the ability to obtain a history is limited in the obtunded patient, inspection for areas of ecchymosis, palpable step-off, or gross malalignment is important. A thorough and systematic neurologic examination may reveal both obvious and subtle deficits. In the unresponsive patient, this may be limited to bulbocavernosus reflex assessment. Distracting injuries, such as extremity fractures, should be taken into consideration when examining for spinal tenderness or neurologic deficits. Initial radiographs should include AP and lateral views of painful regions. In the obtunded patient, AP and lateral radiographs of the cervical, thoracic, and lumbar spine are important to obtain.

Imaging Studies

CT is the advanced imaging modality of choice in the assessment of fractures. CT scans should be obtained of any area with a known or suspected injury. Thin-cut slices from uninjured levels above and below the fracture are also useful. Sagittal and coronal reconstructions aid in fracture visualization and should be a routine part of the trauma study (Figure 1).

MRI is indicated in patients with a neurologic deficit. MRI is also useful for detecting ligamentous injuries, such

FIGURE 1

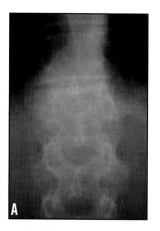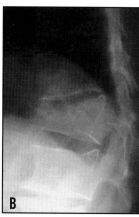

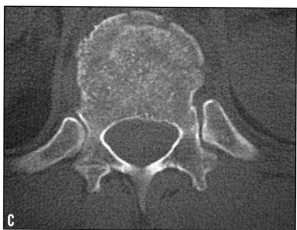

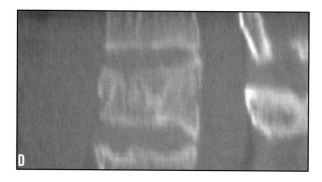

Imaging studies of a 50-year-old man with a T12 compression fracture. Mild posterior gapping is demonstrated on AP **(A)** and lateral **(B)** radiographs. CT scans **(C** and **D)** demonstrate fractures of the superior lip and body.

as disruptions of the posterior ligamentous complex (PLC), that can directly affect the decision whether to treat a fracture nonsurgically or surgically (Figure 2).

History of Nonsurgical Management

The history of nonsurgical management of thoracolumbar fractures dates back to Hippocrates, who reported using methods of postural reduction to treat traumatic deformity. Thousands of years later, in the early twentieth century, similar principles were still being used. In 1935, Bohler[1] proclaimed that a good anatomic result was requisite for a good functional result. In 1938, Watson-Jones[2] maintained a similar focus on restoration of alignment, stating that a "perfect recovery" was possible only if a "perfect reduction" was obtained. Watson-Jones also believed that even small amounts of residual vertebral body wedging could lead to persistent pain. At the time, no reliable method of correction existed for such wedging.

As is a common trend in orthopaedics, efforts were spent developing methods and maneuvers to achieve or at least improve anatomic reduction of thoracolumbar spinal fractures, and the introduction of each new technique reinforced the perceived validity of this approach. Thus, the principle of anatomic fracture alignment gained credence despite the lack of true scientific evidence supporting its efficacy.

Recognizing this, in 1949 Nicoll[3] sought to challenge this unsubstantiated principle, publishing a landmark work that critically analyzed the results of nonsurgical treatment of spinal fractures in a homogeneous group of coal miners with similar injuries. In sharp contradistinction to researchers who concentrated on pain and radiographic parameters, Nicoll assessed functional outcomes by measuring strength and mobility. In addition, unlike most of his contemporaries, he presented results at 5-year follow-up. Through his analysis, Nicoll was the first to distinguish between stable and unstable thoracolumbar fractures.

Nicoll strictly defined a good functional result as a patient being able to return to work without discomfort or disability for at least a 2-year period. Though fractures from other regions were included in the study, most (77%) occurred at the thoracolumbar junction (T11-L2). Most of the fractures were defined as anterior wedge fractures, which most likely would be referred to today as compression fractures. All patients with wedge fractures returned to work, although 28% reported residual pain at the fracture site. Of those treated with a hyperextension plaster cast, 72% reported

FIGURE 2

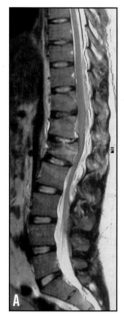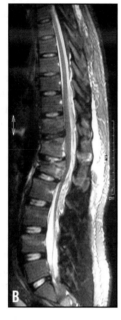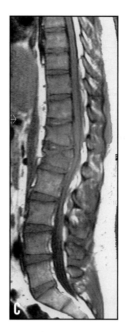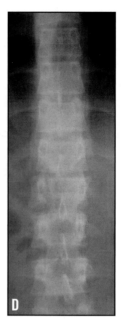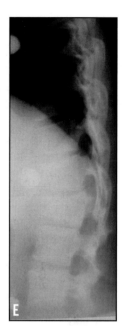

Imaging studies of a 21-year-old construction worker who fell from a ladder. He was neurologically intact and reported only mild back pain. Initial radiographs demonstrated a T12 compression fracture and an L1 burst-type fracture, and a CT scan revealed anteroposterior canal diameter compromise of about 30%. Because the competency of the posterior ligaments was in question, the patient underwent an MRI examination. T2-weighted (**A**) and short time inversion recovery (STIR) (**B**) images demonstrated some mildly increased signal, but the continuity of the interspinous ligaments and the ligamentum flavum did not appear to be disrupted. This was confirmed on T1-weighted images (**C**). The patient was placed in a thoracolumbosacral orthosis and weight-bearing AP (**D**) and lateral (**E**) radiographs were obtained, which demonstrated no increased kyphosis compared with initial radiographs. At 1-week follow-up, the patient reported no back pain. Follow-up radiographs revealed no progression of kyphosis, and the patient remained neurologically intact.

nonspecific low back pain at the lumbosacral junction. Nicoll postulated that prolonged hyperextension might shorten the posterior ligaments, leading to the pain. Patients described symptoms that were mild at rest and increased with sitting, standing, or moderate exercise. Based on these findings, Nicoll believed that such "stable" wedge fractures could be treated with early ambulation and no bracing.

"Other" methods were used to treat 20% of the patients, most often for unstable injuries such as fracture-dislocations. Only 37% reported nonspecific lumbosacral pain. Overall, nearly 40% of patients returned to full duty, with the remainder able to perform light duty. Ten patients had fracture-dislocations and no neurologic deficit; seven of these returned to full duty after plaster cast treatment. Based on his findings, Nicoll recommended that unstable injuries should be treated with a plaster cast to prevent worsening deformity and to protect the spinal cord and should be kept at bed rest for 6 months.

CLASSIFICATION SYSTEMS

The Holdsworth Classification System

Departing from Nicoll, Holdsworth[4,5] proposed that the critical determinant of spinal stability was integrity of the PLC, the posterior column of a two-column spine. In his classic article published in 1963, Holdsworth defined the PLC as the zygoapophyseal articular processes and associated facet capsules, interspinous process ligaments, supraspinous ligaments, and ligamentum flava.[4] Holdsworth also introduced the concept of a mechanistic classification of spinal fractures. He described four types (or mechanisms) of injury: flexion, flexion and rotation, extension, and compression. Based on his experience, Holdsworth observed that rotational injuries frequently led to disruption of the PLC but that pure flexion rarely disrupted it. Pure compression injuries, known today as burst fractures, led to posterior fragment retropulsion into the spinal canal and, in some cases, tearing of the dura and neurologic compromise.

The Denis Classification System

Denis,[6] expanding on the basic two-column mechanistic description of instability, proposed a three-column theory of clinical spinal stability/instability. In Denis's system, the posterior column was the same as in Holdsworth's system; however, the anterior column consisted of the anterior portion of the vertebral body, the anterior longitudinal ligament, and the disk, while the middle column consisted of the posterior vertebral body, the posterior longitudinal ligament, and the disk. Denis made this distinction to highlight the importance of the middle column, which he believed to be critical for spinal stability. One potential weakness of his theory, however, is that some, if not most, burst-type fractures are mechanically stable and can be successfully treated nonsurgically.[7-10] The Denis classification system is described more fully in chapter 3.

REPORTED RESULTS

Nonsurgical Treatment of Stable Fractures in Patients Without Neurologic Deficit

Young[11] reported on a series of 623 patients with thoracolumbar fractures defined as stable, based on Holdsworth's two-column theory. He found that at 3- to 8-year follow-up, 75% were able to return to work, of whom half returned to light duty, and 25% were unable to work because of pain. Degenerative changes and deformity were found to a similar degree in patients who were symptom-free as in those with symptoms.

Weinstein and associates[12] reported the results of nonsurgical treatment of "stable" thoracolumbar burst fractures with bone retropulsion in 42 patients without neurologic deficit who were followed for 11 to 55 years. Treatment ranged from body casts and mobilization to 3 months of bed rest. Though average kyphosis was 26° in flexion and 17° in extension, the degree of kyphosis did not correlate with degree of pain or function at final follow-up. No neurologic deterioration was reported. Low back pain scores, averaging 3.5 on the visual analog scale, were reported, with no patient using narcotics for pain control, and 88% of patients returned to work in their preinjury occupation.

Folman and Gepstein[8] reviewed the records of 85 patients treated nonsurgically for thoracolumbar wedge fractures with at least 3 years' follow-up. The exact treatment regimen was not detailed, but it was specified that some patients received physiotherapy and/or brace treatment. The authors reported a 69% incidence of nonspecific chronic low back pain, which was similar to Nicoll's[3] findings. In contrast to Weinstein and associates'[12] findings, the degree of kyphosis correlated with pain intensity, although no critical value of kyphosis was defined. Loss of vertebral body height did not correlate with outcome, nor did use of bracing or physiotherapy.

Shen and Shen[7] retrospectively reviewed outcomes of nonsurgical treatment of 38 patients with thoracolumbar burst fractures with no neurologic deficit. Exclusion criteria included injuries with posterior arch fractures, dislocations, or kyphosis greater than 35°. Only nine patients were treated in a brace; all were permitted early ambulation. Average kyphosis increased from 20° to 24° at an average follow-up of 4 years. Thirty-two patients reported either no pain or mild pain; four had moderate pain; and two patients, both of whom underwent surgery more than 1 year after injury, had severe pain. No correlation was found between kyphosis or spinal canal compromise and clinical outcome. Twenty-nine patients returned to their preinjury occupation. Complications included transient hematuria and urinary retention, which occurred in three and six patients, respectively.

Aligizakis and associates[9] followed, for an average of 42 months, 60 consecutive neurologically intact patients with thoracolumbar fractures treated with an orthosis. Initial and final kyphosis averaged 6° and 8°, respectively. The functional outcome was satisfactory in 55 patients (91%). Fifty patients (83%) reported no or slight pain and were able to return to preinjury activity levels. Urinary tract infections developed in three patients and were treated successfully with antibiotics.

Studies Comparing Nonsurgical and Surgical Treatment

The results of surgical and nonsurgical treatment have been compared in select groups of patients with clearly defined thoracolumbar injuries. Shen and associates[13] prospectively compared outcomes of patients with thoracolumbar burst fractures and no neurologic deficit who were either treated with posterior surgery or managed nonsurgically. Injuries that involved the posterior arch, such as facet dislocations, were excluded. In the 47 patients managed nonsurgically, treatment consisted of a hyperextension brace and early ambulation. In the 33 patients treated with surgery, short segment pedicle screw fixation and fusion was used. Outcome scores were better in the surgical group at 3 months, but no statistically significant differences were noted at 6-month and 2-year follow-up. Kyphosis correction was initially better in the surgical group, but this advantage was lost with time. Pain scores followed a similar pattern.

More recently, Wood and associates[10] published results of a prospective, randomized, controlled study comparing surgical and nonsurgical treatment of thoracolumbar burst fractures in patients without neurologic deficit. Importantly, they excluded injuries with suspected or confirmed posterior ligamentous disruption. Nonsurgical care included a brace or cast followed by early mobilization. Surgical treatment was by either anterior or posterior surgical stabilization. No statistical differences were found with respect to kyphosis, functional outcome scores, or pain, although surgically treated patients tended to have higher pain scores. Complications were more common in the surgical group.

These studies strongly suggest that nonsurgical management consisting of bracing and early mobilization is effective for stable thoracolumbar burst fractures, defined as fractures without substantial posterior ligamentous injury (Figure 3). Neither study, however, provided clear criteria to distinguish between stable and unstable burst fractures.

Nonsurgical Treatment of "Unstable" Fractures

Defining stability according to the Denis system, Chow and associates[14] reported the results of nonsurgical treatment of 24 neurologically intact patients with "unstable" burst fractures. All of the patients had fractures that involved the anterior and the middle columns, and none had lamina or facet fractures. Ten had evidence of interspinous widening consistent with a posterior ligamentous disruption. The mean kyphosis at the fracture site was 5.3° (range, 11° lordosis to 20° kyphosis). Treatment consisted of thoracolumborsacral orthoses, Jewett hyperextension braces (three-point braces that apply pressure at the sternum and pelvis anteriorly and have a strap posteriorly, preventing flexion), or hyperextension casts and early ambulation. No patient had a neurologic deficit, and 18 returned to work. Of the nine patients with a posterior ligamentous injury still alive at final follow-up, all had returned to work. A statistically insignificant increase in kyphosis was observed, similar to Shen and Shen's[7] findings.

FIGURE 3

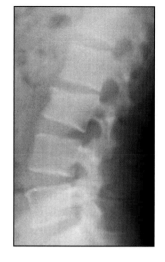

Lateral radiograph demonstrating a simple L3 compression in a 20-year-old man with a 1-week history of back pain after a fall while snowboarding off a mogul. The pain resolved completely after 3 months of activity modification without bracing. Follow-up radiographs demonstrated no kyphotic progression.

Willen and associates[15] compared the results of surgical versus nonsurgical management of unstable thoracolumbar fractures in a group of neurologically intact patients. The average hospital stay was significantly longer for the patients treated nonsurgically (80 days) than for those undergoing surgical treatment (30 days), and average duration of immobilization was longer in the nonsurgical patients (67 days) than in the surgical patients (18 days). Final kyphosis was greater in the nonsurgical patients, but the degree of deformity did not affect functional outcomes. No patient had neurologic deterioration. There was no difference in pain scores or rates of return to work.

According to these data, the main benefit of surgical treatment appears to be earlier mobilization in patients with unstable fractures. However, the risk of secondary neurologic compromise, though low, remains a concern for most practitioners.

Nonsurgical Treatment in the Neurologically Impaired Patient

Though rarely indicated, a nonsurgical approach may sometimes be used to treat fractures in patients with neurologic deficits. This would most commonly be indicated in patients with a complete spinal cord injury who are medically unfit to undergo surgery. In support of this, Dedrinos and associates[16] found that no patient with a thoracolumbar burst fracture associated with a complete injury (Frankel grade A injury) demonstrated neurologic recovery, regardless of whether surgical or nonsurgical treatment was used. A 5° reduction in kyphosis was associated with recovery of one nerve root level and/or one Frankel grade, regardless of the treatment method used. Similarly, Burke and Murray[17] reviewed the results of nonsurgical management of 89 patients with thoracolumbar injuries and neurologic compromise, compared with 26 treated surgically. Neurologic recovery was documented in 35% of the patients treated nonsurgically and 38% of the patients treated surgically.

Role of Spinal Canal Compromise

The severity of spinal canal compromise appears to have little influence on the incidence or prognosis of neurologic impairment after thoracolumbar fractures. Patients with similar canal compromise can differ widely in neurologic status. Furthermore, insufficient evidence exists to demonstrate that canal decompression improves neural recovery,[18,19] even though decompression is commonly performed. Nearly equivalent canal remodeling occurs with both nonsurgical management and surgical management (ie, indirect reduction).[20]

SUMMARY AND CONCLUSIONS

Although various reports have demonstrated good results with nonsurgical treatment of thoracolumbar fractures, it should not be inferred that nonsurgical treatment is appropriate for every injury. Various factors must be taken into account, including fracture stability, neurologic status, associated injuries, comorbidities, and patient reliability.

Our practice is to surgically treat injuries that are clearly unstable, regardless of neurologic status. Associated injuries such as severe chest contusions and pneumothorax or hemothorax that require chest tubes, which might preclude effective brace treatment, are potential indications (or considerations) for surgical management. We prefer to treat patients with a neurologic deficit surgically in order to decompress the neural elements if necessary and to stabilize the spinal column to maximize the opportunities to recover function and/or prevent deterioration. For those who have significant canal compromise and can tolerate the procedure, an anterior approach is used. Posterolateral decompression is also a reasonable option but is associated with greater blood loss. When neural deficit is present without significant canal compromise or the patient has a complete spinal cord injury, posterior instrumentation and fusion is usually adequate and preferred.

Nonsurgical management is preferred for most simple compression fractures, provided the PLC is intact. Kyphosis greater than 30° to 35°, substantial loss of anterior vertebral body height (more than 40% to 50%), or interspinous process gapping strongly suggest posterior ligamentous disruption. If the integrity of the PLC is in question, MRI of the thoracolumbar junction can provide useful information.

Our approach to treatment of a thoracolumbar burst fracture in a neurologically intact patient depends on an assessment of stability, which, unfortunately, can be quite challenging. Many criteria have been proposed, but we believe that fractures with more than 25° of segmental kyphosis, facet or spinous process gapping, or CT or MRI evidence of PLC disruption should be considered unstable, in which case surgical management should be considered.

In acute injuries that do not fulfill these criteria for instability but do have some increased kyphosis and/or a burst component, bed rest and logrolling precautions are maintained until a custom thoracolumbosacral orthosis is fit. After ambulation is initiated, AP and lateral radiographs are obtained with the patient standing in the brace. If alignment is maintained, ambulation can continue. Radiographs should be obtained at frequent intervals for 1 year after the brace is removed. We educate patients to be alert to the symptoms of conus medullaris or cauda equina compression, including fecal/urinary retention or incontinence and sensorimotor changes. If a new neurologic deficit (extremity weakness or increasing numbness) develops, additional radiographs, CT, and MRI should be obtained, and surgery may be indicated. Persistent subacute or late pain that correlates with the fracture site is also a possible indication for surgical management.

Compression fractures without significant kyphosis or bone retropulsion, usually those with mild anterior wedging or axial compression, can be treated with a Jewett brace to help control flexion and decrease rotation. Often these injuries heal early. Isometric abdominal and back strengthening exercises and general aerobic conditioning can begin at 6 to 8 weeks after the injury.

REFERENCES

1. Bohler L: *Treatment of Fractures*. Bristol, England, John Wright and Son, 1935.
2. Watson-Jones R: The results of postural reduction of fractures of the spine. *J Bone Joint Surg Am* 1938;20:567-586.

3. Nicoll EA: Fractures of the dorso-lumbar spine. *J Bone Joint Surg Br* 1949;31:376-394.

4. Holdsworth FW: Fractures, dislocations, and fracture-dislocations of the spine. *J Bone Joint Surg Br* 1963;45:6-20.

5. Holdsworth FW: Fractures, dislocations, and fracture-dislocations of the spine. *J Bone Joint Surg Am* 1970;52:1534-1551.

6. Denis F: The three column spine and its significance in the classification of acute thoracolumbar spinal injuries. *Spine* 1983;8:817-831.

7. Shen WJ, Shen YS: Non-surgical treatment of three-column thoracolumbar junction burst fractures without neurologic deficit. *Spine* 1999;24:412-415.

8. Folman Y, Gepstein R: Late outcome of nonoperative management of thoracolumbar vertebral wedge fractures. *J Orthop Trauma* 2003;17:190-192.

9. Aligizakis A, Katonis P, Stergiopoulos K, Galanakis I, Karabekios S, Hadjipavlou A: Functional outcome of burst fractures of the thoracolumbar spine managed non-operatively with early ambulation, evaluated using the load sharing classification. *Acta Orthop Belg* 2002;68:279-287.

10. Wood K, Butterman G, Mehbod A, Garvey T, Jhanjee R, Sechriest V: Operative compared with nonoperative treatment of a thoracolumbar burst fracture without neurological deficit. *J Bone Joint Surg* 2003;85-A:773-781.

11. Young MH: Long-term consequences of stable fractures of the thoracic and lumbar vertebral bodies. *J Bone Joint Surg Br* 1973;55:295-300.

12. Weinstein JN, Collalto P, Lehmann TR: Thoracolumbar "burst" fractures treated conservatively: A long-term follow-up. *Spine* 1988;13:33-38.

13. Shen WJ, Liu TJ, Shen YS: Nonoperative treatment versus posterior fixation for thoracolumbar junction burst fractures without neurologic deficit. *Spine* 2001;26:1038-1045.

14. Chow GH, Nelson BJ, Beghard JS, Brugman JL, Brown CW, Donaldson DH: Functional outcome of thoracolumbar burst fractures managed with hyperextension casting or bracing and early mobilization. *Spine* 1996;21:2170-2175.

15. Willen J, Lindahl S, Nordwall A: Unstable thoracolumbar fractures: A comparative clinical study of conservative treatment and Harrington instrumentation. *Spine* 1985;10:111-122.

16. Dedrinos GK, Halikias JG, Krallis PN, Asimakopoulos A: Factors influencing neurological recovery in burst thoracolumbar fractures. *Acta Orthop Belg* 1995;61:226-234.

17. Burke DC, Murray DD: The management of thoracic and thoracolumbar injuries of the spine with neurological involvement. *J Bone Joint Surg Br* 1976;58:72-78.

18. Boerger TO, Limb D, Dickson RA: Does 'canal clearance' affect neurological outcome after thoracolumbar burst fractures? *J Bone Joint Surg Br* 2000;82:629-635.

19. Vaccaro AR, Nachwalter RS, Klein GR, Sewards JM, Albert TJ, Garfin SR: The significance of thoracolumbar spinal canal size in spinal cord injury patients. *Spine* 2001;26:371-376.

20. Dai LY: Remodeling of the spinal canal after thoracolumbar burst fractures. *Clin Orthop* 2001;382:119-123.

CHAPTER 7

IMPLANT ALTERNATIVES IN SURGICAL MANAGEMENT

RAMAN DHAWAN, MD
BRUCE E. FREDRICKSON, MD
HANSEN A. YUAN, MD

The thoracolumbar region is a transitional area of the spine; a concentration of forces occurs in this region during trauma, making it more susceptible to injury and persistent instability following trauma. Most spinal injuries occur following a combination of flexion and axial compression and/or distraction. In a multicenter review of more than 1,000 patients with spine fractures, 52% of injuries occurred at the thoracolumbar junction.[1] Nearly half of these injuries are the result of motor vehicle accidents; the rest occur as a result of a variety of causes, principally falls, sports activities, and trauma due to violence.[2] Males between the ages of 10 and 40 are at highest risk. Significant three-column injuries may result in neurologic deficit.[3] Many of these result in unstable injuries that require surgical stabilization and early mobilization.

Controversies persist regarding the indications for the appropriate surgical approach: posterior, anterior, or circumferential. Regardless of the surgical approach or the instrumentation, however, the main considerations for any surgical treatment of thoracolumbar injuries remain the same: (1) anatomic reduction of the fracture; (2) rigid fixation; (3) neural decompression, when necessary; (4) early mobilization and rehabilitation; and (5) a functional, painless spinal column.

GENERAL PRINCIPLES OF SPINE FIXATION

When selecting a fixation system that will stabilize the injured spine, both the damaged structures and the structures that can still support load must be considered. In general, the primary function of the disk-vertebra complex is to resist compression, shear, and torsion. The facets control rotation and prevent anteroposterior shearing. The posterior ligaments and facets prevent excessive flexion and lateral bending. With this in mind, it is possible to select instrumentation appropriate to the type of injury.

The most important biomechanical consideration for the use of implants in spinal trauma is that the strength of the particular system should ideally match the instabilities of the injury. For example, a flexion-distraction injury in which the fulcrum is anterior to the anterior aspect of the vertebral body may damage the posterior ligaments, spinous processes, facet capsules or pedicles, disk, and vertebra. The affected motion segment can resist compressive and shear load but not excessive flexion. For these injuries, tension band instrumentation, consisting of wires passed around the spinous processes, pedicle screws, facet screws, or compressive hook-rod systems, can be used for fixation (Figure 1).

A compressive force combined with flexion can damage the posterior elements and cause the anterior part of the vertebra to collapse. In this situation, the posterior disk and vertebral wall act as the fulcrum (the fulcrum is in the middle column). This type of injury reduces the stability of the spine, and depending on the condition of the anterior longitudinal ligament, instrumentation may need to support both compression and tension (distraction) (Figure 2).

With injuries caused primarily by compressive loading, characterized by loss of both anterior and posterior vertebral body height and facet or pedicle fracture but with

FIGURE 1

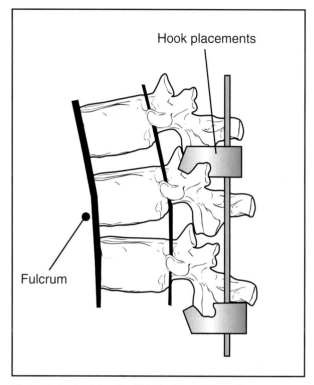

Flexion-distraction injury in which the fulcrum is anterior to the vertebral body.

FIGURE 2

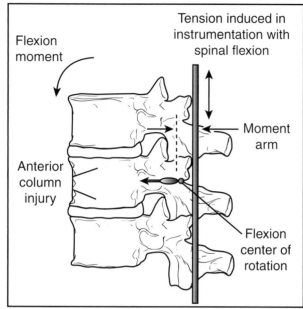

Anterior-posterior column injury in which the fulcrum is in the middle column.

intact anterior and posterior ligaments, the affected motion segment will not resist compression and shear adequately. The loss of vertebral body height reduces tension in the surrounding ligaments, which decreases resistance to flexion, extension, and rotation (Figure 3). To restore flexion and extension and compressive stability, vertebral body height must be restored. In these situations, very stable instrumentation is required. The compressive load must be borne by either an interbody device or by a device fixed to the posterior aspect of the vertebrae that can resist cantilever forces.

A fracture created by torsional loading typically injures the facets and the vertebral body so that the spinal motion segment may resist compression adequately but not shear and torsion. Parallel instrumentation attached to the posterior lamina of two vertebrae by hooks, wires, or pedicle screws results in a four-bar linkage, which does not adequately resist torsional loads.[4] Adding a cross link between the longitudinal rods will increase torsional stiffness[5] (Figure 4).

THE POSTERIOR BONE-IMPLANT INTERFACE

The ability of an implant to transfer load in different directions and magnitudes depends on the bone-implant interface. With posterior instrumentation, the lamina, transverse process, or in the case of pedicle screw attachment, the vertebral body, are the sites at which load is transferred. The lamina is the strongest purchase site of the posterior spine and the least affected by osteoporosis.[6] The pullout (direct posterior loading) strength of the lamina is highest for the lumbar spine and lowest for the midthoracic spine.[7] The transverse process is the weakest point of hook attachment. The lumbar lamina is significantly stronger than the thoracic lamina. The hook-lamina interface transfers load only in compression between the bone and hook material. Pivoting occurs between the hook and lamina so that the hook does not directly control flexion rotation of the vertebra (Figure 5). The interaction of the rod with the lamina can prevent flexion rotation. This can be augmented by the addition of rod sleeves or by the use of sublaminar wires.

Sublaminar wiring is not effective in transmitting axial loads to the rods, and slippage of wires on rods can occur

FIGURE 3

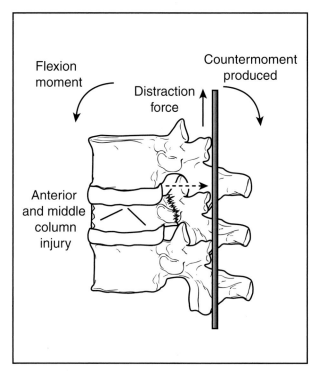

Compressive loading resulting in loss of both anterior and posterior vertebral body height. The posterior device resists cantilever forces.

FIGURE 4

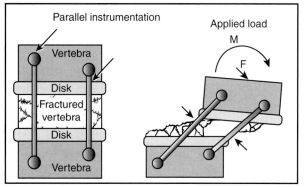

Parallel instrumentation consisting of two rods fixed by screws can become an unstable linkage, allowing shortening and shearing of an unstable motion segment. Use of a coupler to produce an H configuration can prevent this effect.

THE ANTERIOR BONE-IMPLANT INTERFACE

Anteriorly there are two ways to attach an implant to the vertebral body. First, some anterior implants are simply interposed between adjacent vertebrae without secure mechanical attachment. These implants articulate between the device and the end plate to provide stability. They may resist shear and rotation somewhat, depending on the interface between the device and the end plates. Direct contact between the vertebral end plate and the implant is weakest in compression in the center and strongest at the periphery.[11] Thus, most of the contact should be at the periphery. A typical interbody construct does not resist extension. After incorporation of a bone graft or bone growth into the metal and the implant, the interbody load-bearing capacity is substantially improved (Figure 7). Interbody implants can include autograft or allograft struts or a variety of cage devices.

The second type of anterior instrumentation device is basically a load-sharing implant. These implants should be placed along the lateral aspect of the anterior column to avoid applying pressure on the great vessels. The vertebral screws need to be directed in a triangular configuration to provide maximum resistance to pullout. Resistance to pullout is superior with bicortical screw purchase. The anterior instrumentation devices rely directly on load transmission through an interbody construct placed simultaneously. The status of the posterior vertebral complex also must be considered when anterior instrumenta-

during lateral bending, flexion, and compression loading.[5] The hook-rod assembly has the best posterior loading strength compared with double or single wires.[8] Single wire in particular tends to cut through or fail at a much lower load than double wires or hook systems.

Pedicle screws are an alternative to fixation by hooks or wires. This type of fixation permits the transmission of moments in all directions, except about the axis of the screw. The pullout strength of pedicle screws depends on the shear strength of the cancellous bone into which it is embedded and the area of shear force. Thus, the larger the diameter of the screw and greater its depth, the greater is the pullout strength and resistance to cyclic loading failure.[9,10]

Pedicle screw fixation is best at the level of the pedicle. The soft cancellous bone anteriorly may allow toggling of the screw when the forces applied exceed the strength of bone. Extension of the pedicle screw into the subcortical bone of the anterior vertebral body will help prevent this phenomenon (Figure 6).

FIGURE 5

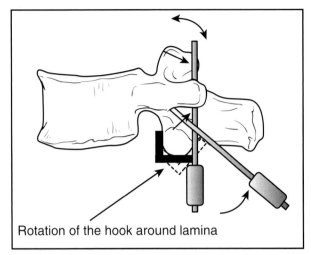

Rotation of the hook around lamina

Nonparallel configuration prevents shear and shortening of the motion segment.

FIGURE 6

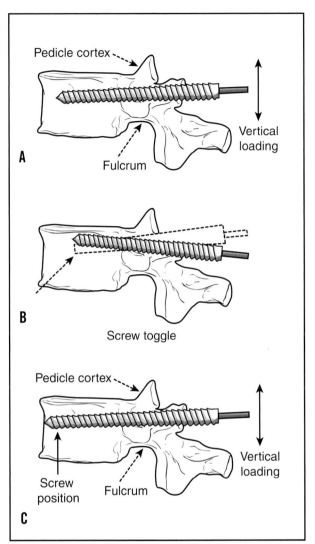

A, Ideal position of pedicle screw, placed in subcortical bone. **B,** Screws that are too short may result in toggling. **C,** Screws that are too long may result in injury to anterior structures such as vascular structures.

tion is used (Figure 8). In the presence of posterior instability, anterior instrumentation alone tends to fail.

SPINAL CONSTRUCTS

The torso's center of gravity is anterior to the spine. Flexion and compression are the predominant modes of loading. For the same applied moment, an instrumentation system with multiple attachments over a large number of spinal motion segments will produce smaller forces at the implant-bone interface[5] (Figure 9). The use of parallel rods without cross links allows the implant to act as a four-bar linkage. This permits torsion, lateral bending, and lateral shear for posteriorly applied instrumentation. Alternatively, for anterior fixation, this allows flexion, extension, and anteroposterior shear.[5] Orienting the pedicle screws so that the axes of rotation are not parallel, the use of cross links, or attachment to at least three vertebral levels helps prevent this effect.[4] Pedicular fixation to the vertebrae adjacent to the fractured vertebra with the anterior column injury results in large screw forces. These forces can be reduced, however, by increasing the length of the moment arm, by distributing the forces over a greater number of screws, or by using an anterior support. In addition, viscoelastic creep of the soft tissue of spine will decrease the distractive force over a period of time, resulting in lower forces of purchase at the lamina.[5,12]

POSTERIOR INSTRUMENTATION SYSTEMS

The relative indications for posterior instrumentation are broad and include treating neurologically intact patients with unstable fractures or patients with neurologic deficits and canal compromise. Posterior instrumentation can perform an indirect closed reduction by ligamentotaxis.[13]

FIGURE 7

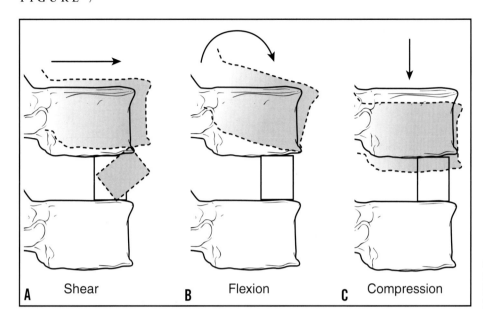

Anterior interbody implant. Lack of secure attachment results in shear (**A**) and flexion (**B**). End plates resist compression (**C**).

FIGURE 8

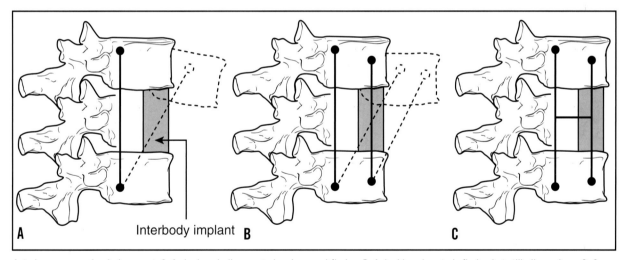

Anterior screws and rod placement. **A,** A single rod allows anterior shear and flexion. **B,** A double rod controls flexion but still allows shear. **C,** Cross linkage prevents both.

Harrington Rod Instrumentation

Harrington rod instrumentation was the first effective system for the treatment of thoracolumbar fractures. The rods apply a progressive reduction force in a single plane, either axial distraction or axial compression. Harrington rods provide rotational correction only by a combination of forces created between hook-lamina and rod-lamina contact. To be effective, Harrington rods require intact longitudinal ligaments and instrumentation two to three levels above and below the injury. Contouring Harrington rods or adding sleeves allows application of both a distraction force and extension moment to correct traumatic kyphosis. Segmental fixation with sublaminar wires, as applied to Luque rods or to Harrington rods,

FIGURE 9

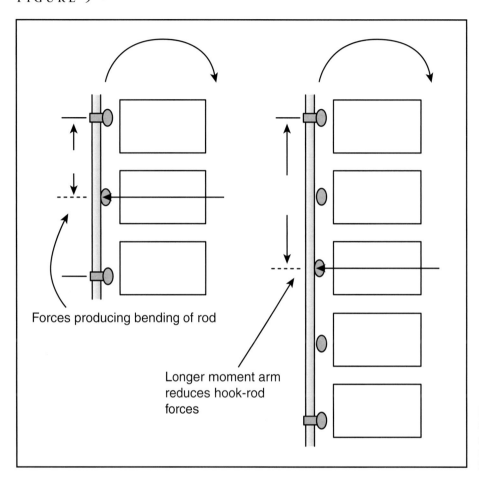

Forces producing bending of rod

Longer moment arm
reduces hook-rod
forces

Biomechanical comparison of short
(A) and long **(B)** rods. Longer constructs reduce hook-rod forces because of the larger moment arm of
the rod.

provides poor control of axial height but increases rotational stability. The rod-sleeve construct imparts a degree of rotational stability because the sleeves wedge between the facets and spinous processes. The rod-sleeve technique, similar to a pure hook-rod-sleeve system, does not provide adequate stabilization for shear injuries.

Segmental Hook-Rod Methods

Segmental hook-rod methods, including Cotrel-Dubousset (Medtronics Sofamor Danek, Memphis, TN), Texas Scottish Rite Hospital (Medtronics Sofamor Danek), and ISOLA (DePuy Spine, Raynham, MA), are useful in many spinal injury patterns. The system uses segmental fixation with hooks or screws, allowing the hooks to be placed on the same rod simultaneously, in distraction or compression. After all the hooks are in place, distraction forces can be

applied to the rod to relieve axial compression. The rods can be prebent or bent in situ to reduce the kyphotic deformity. The rotational stability with the segmental hook-rod method is good, especially when cross-linking devices are used. For increased correction of kyphotic deformities, stiffer rods, which will better resist flexion forces, are available. The disadvantage of segmental fixation is the increased length of instrumentation. Attempts to shorten the instrumentation by applying two hooks at the same lamina have resulted in higher failure rate.[14]

Pedicle Screw Fixation

Pedicle screws provide a strong anchor to the spine, resulting in shorter constructs in fracture fixation. Pedicle screw fixation directly controls the three columns of the spine, provides four-point fixation, and allows short constructs. Three-vertebrae, two-motion-segment fixation is feasible and avoids unnecessary sacrifice of the uninjured motion segments. Stronger corrective forces can be applied to the injured segment than with other techniques.

The accurate placement of pedicle screws above T10 becomes increasingly difficult. The pedicles are narrow; therefore, smaller pedicle screws are required. A thorough knowledge of pedicle dimensions and size is crucial for the safe application of screw fixation. Smaller screws (less than 6-mm diameter) are not strong enough to withstand the loads and are subject to fatigue failure. Short segment pedicle screw constructs a single level above and below the fracture at the thoracolumbar junction may be inadequate to correct and withstand the applied forces in some patients with small pedicles. The excessive bending force applied to the screws has resulted in frequent screw failure, bending, and device loosening.

Pedicle screw systems with plate fixation are also available. The classic design is that of Roy-Camille. The plates, perforated with holes at 13-mm intervals for screw placement, are precontoured and designed for use in the thoracic and lumbar spines. The system is a four-point device, immobilizing normal motion segments above and below the lesion.

The external fixator Magerl[15] developed in 1984 for stabilization of spine fractures used Schantz pedicular screws. This fixator allows fracture reduction while immobilizing one level above and one level below the injured vertebra. In 1987, Dick[16] modified the external fixator to the internal fixator, a fully implantable system. It originally consisted of 5-mm Schantz screws placed into the pedicle and 7-mm flattened rods that connected to the pedicle screws. The unit connecting the Schantz screws to the rod is mobile and allows application of sequentially separate reduction forces in two planes, specifically kyphosis or lordosis and distraction or compression. The Schantz screws are long and provide a strong lever arm that helps during fracture reduction. The diameter of these screws has been increased to 6 mm because the 5-mm screws were known to fail. Comparing the pullout strength, displacement, and energy absorption before failure of several pedicle screw designs in human cadaveric vertebrae, the 6-mm screw had greater pullout strength.[17] Multiple pedicle systems are currently available and can be used for fracture fixation. The ease of use while attempting fracture reduction is an important consideration.

ANTERIOR SURGICAL APPROACH

The favored surgical approach to the spine traditionally has been posterior. Failure to achieve canal clearance by posterior instrumentation techniques using ligamentotaxis and/or open posterior decompression may necessitate a more direct approach for decompression—the anterior approach.

With the anterior approach, the spinal cord is under direct visualization. Associated nerve root injuries can be evaluated and/or decompressed. In patients with multiple traumatic injuries, retroperitoneal and intraperitoneal injuries can be repaired through the same incision. Complete decompression of the fracture fragments impinging on the dural sac is facilitated.

Most early reports described anterior cord decompression and bone grafting without instrumentation.[18] Failure of these constructs led to the development of anterior fixation devices. Anterior instrumentation devices are load-sharing implants; thus, meticulous care is required when sizing and shaping the bone graft. The anterior instrumentation and interbody construct work together and require precise balance of the devices. This technique establishes stability by tensioning the paravertebral ligaments and provides resistance to compressive loads by placement of a graft of the correct size.[11]

The vertebral screws need to be directed in a triangular configuration to provide maximum resistance to pullout. Failure to provide firm compression of the graft will result in construct failure.

Milgram designed the first anterior device for anterior spine fixation in 1953.[18] Used for kyphosis correction, this device was not successful. In the late 1960s, Dwyer[19] was the first to popularize an anterior spinal fixation system for scoliosis. Dunn[20] introduced an anterior distraction fixation and fusion device for thoracolumbar spine fractures in the mid 1980s, a biomechanically sound device that was able to withstand both axial and rotational loading. However, several fatal aortic and common iliac vessel aneurysms were reported secondary to erosion of the vessels caused by these implants. The Kostuik-Harrington device combined a Harrington distraction rod in front and a compression hook farther back clamped to the vertebra by specially modified bone screws.[21] The device did not attain widespread popularity despite excellent results reported.

Kaneda and associates[22] developed a system that allowed graft compression. Paravertebral rods allow direct dynamic distraction of the vertebrae to ease exposure of the end plates and dura, followed by direct compression of implanted bone graft after decompression of the neural elements. The device is extremely rigid once inserted. The principal disadvantage is that the bone screws and connecting rods are prominent, which may increase the danger of vessel injury, especially if the implant is placed anteriorly. Additionally, the rigidity of the device may promote unwanted stress shielding in the instrumented vertebrae and bone graft.

In contrast to these bulky devices, which allow direct compression of the bone graft, plate systems have been developed for anterior application to the thoracolumbar spine. Black and associates[23] introduced a multiple-hole low-profile contoured plate for lateral placement on the vertebral body.

Yuan and associates[24] developed the Syracuse I-Plate, a plate that is 3 mm thick and angulated so that 60° of curvature separate the two adjacent screw holes. The plate is applied with two screws inserted into the intact vertebral bodies above and below the injured vertebra. The rigidity of the I-plate was compared with the Kostuik-Harrington construct and the Kaneda device (Depuy Spine) in a burst fracture model (KA Mann, MD, and associates, unpublished data, 1987). All but the Kostuik-Harrington system, which was less stable in flexion, improved spinal stability. All were stable in extension. Mann and asssociates[25] compared the I-Plate to the Dick device, concluding that the I-plate was more stable in axial rotation than the Dick device when the posterior elements were intact. However, when the posterior vertebral complex was compromised, the I-plate was less stable. The authors also concluded that the I-Plate was inadequate to stabilize a burst fracture model with posterior disruption. This conclusion applied to all anterior instrumentation systems.

Summary and Conclusions

There is no "best" instrumentation system; each device has its merits and disadvantages. Surgeons should use a system with which they have gained familiarity and which they feel comfortable using to treat complex injuries and deformities. Like internal fixation of long bone fractures, internal fixation of spine fractures is a legitimate, valid treatment option. Surgical management of thoracolumbar fractures has numerous advantages: (1) it enables reduction of the fracture/deformity; (2) it allows decompression, either direct or indirect, of the neural canal; (3) it provides stabilization; and (4) it minimizes bracing and allows for safe, early mobilization.

Anterior instrumentation, in conjunction with bone grafting, is sufficient to sustain physiologic loads when the posterior column is intact. With disruption of the posterior complex, however, posterior stabilization is recommended as well. Posterior stabilization alone is satisfactory for most spinal injuries as long as the biomechanics of the injury are well understood and the features of the instrumentation address these biomechanical weaknesses.

References

1. Gertzbein SD: Scoliosis Research Society: Multicenter spine fracture study. *Spine* 1992;17:528-540.
2. Price C, Makintubee S, Herndon W, Istre GR: Epidemiology of traumatic spinal cord injury and acute hospitalization and rehabilitation charges for spinal cord injuries in Oklahoma, 1988-1990. *Am J Epidemiol* 1994;139:37-47.
3. Bohlman HH: Treatment of fractures and dislocations of the thoracic and lumbar spine. *J Bone Joint Surg Am* 1985;67:165-169.
4. Gaines RW, Carson WL, Satterlee CC, et al: Experimental evaluation of seven different fracture internal fixation devices using nonfailure stability testing: The load-sharing and unstable-mechanism concepts. *Spine* 1991;16:902-909.
5. Krag MH: Biomechanics of thoracolumbar spinal fixation: A review. *Spine* 1991;16(suppl):84-99.
6. Coe JD, Herzig MA, Warden KE, et al: Load to failure strengths of spinal implants in osteoporotic spines: A comparison study of pedicle screws, laminar hooks, and spinous process wires. *Trans Orthop Res Soc* 1989;14:71.
7. Tencer AF, Self J, Allen BL Jr, et al: Design and evaluation of a posterior laminar clamp spinal fixation system. *Spine* 1991;16:910-918.
8. McNeice G: Biomechanics research of fracture fixation: Application to the thoracolumbar spine, in *Biomechanics Laboratory Research Report*. Galveston, TX, University of Texas Medical Branch, 1983.
9. Moran JM, Berg WS, Berry JL, et al: Transpedicular screw fixation. *J Orthop Res* 1989;7:107-114.
10. Zindrick MR, Wiltse LL, Widell EH, et al: A biomechanical study of interpeduncular screw fixation in the lumbosacral spine. *Clin Orthop* 1986;203:99-112.
11. Gurr KR, McAfee PC, Shih CM: Biomechanical analysis of anterior and posterior instrumentation systems after corpectomy: A calf-spine model. *J Bone Joint Surg Am* 1988;70:1182-1191.

12. Nagel DA, Edwards WT, Schneider E: Biomechanics of spinal fixation and fusion. *Spine* 1991;16:S151-S154.

13. Crutcher JP Jr, Anderson PA, King HA, et al: Indirect spinal canal decompression in patients with thoracolumbar burst fractures treated by posterior distractive rods. *J Spinal Disord* 1991;4:39-48.

14. McBridge GG: Cotrel-Dubousset rods in surgical stabilization of spinal fractures. *Spine* 1993;18:466-473.

15. Magerl FP: Stabilization of the lower thoracic and lumbar spine with external fixation. *Clin Orthop* 1984;189:125-141.

16. Dick W: The 'fixator interne' as a versatile implant for spine surgery. *Spine* 1987;12:882-900.

17. Skinner R, Transfeldt EE, Maybee J, Venter R, Chalmas W: Experimental pullout testing and comparison of variables in transpedicular screw fixation: A biomechanical study. *Spine* 1990;15:195-201.

18. Kostuik JP: Anterior techniques of stabilization in thoracic and lumbar trauma, in Errico JJ, Bauer RD, Waugh T (eds): *Spinal Trauma*. Philadelphia, PA, Lippincott, 1991, p 282.

19. Dwyer AF: Experience of anterior correction of scoliosis. *Clin Orthop* 1973;93:191-214.

20. Dunn HK: Anterior stabilization of thoracolumbar injuries. *Clin Orthop* 1984;189:116-124.

21. Kostuik JP: Anterior fixation for burst fractures of the thoracic and lumbar spine with or without neurologic involvement. *Spine* 1988;13:286-293.

22. Kaneda K, Abumi K, Fujiya M: Burst fractures with neurologic deficits of the thoracolumbar-lumbar spine: Results of anterior decompression and stabilization with anterior instrumentation. *Spine* 1984;9:788-795.

23. Black RC, Gardner VO, Armstrong GWD, et al: A contoured anterior spinal fixation plate. *Clin Orthop* 1988;227:135-142.

24. Yuan HA, Mann KA, Found EM, et al: Early clinical experience with the Syracuse I-Plate: An anterior spinal fixation device. *Spine* 1988;13:278-285.

25. Mann KA, McGowan DP, Fredrickson BE, Falahee M, Yuan HA: A biomechanical investigation of short segment spinal fixation for burst fracture with varying degrees of posterior disruption. *Spine* 1990;15:470-473.

CHAPTER 8

SURGICAL TREATMENT OF THORACOLUMBAR FRACTURES — POSTERIOR APPROACH

CARLO BELLABARBA, MD

SOHAIL K. MIRZA, MD

JENS R. CHAPMAN, MD

The thoracolumbar region is highly susceptible to injury given its transitional nature at the junction of the mobile lumbar and relatively rigid thoracic spines. Options for treatment of fractures in this area include both nonsurgical and surgical approaches; with the latter, anterior, posterior, or combined approaches are possible. This chapter presents the rationale, the technique, and the relative advantages and disadvantages of the posterior approach to treating thoracolumbar fractures.

Comprehensive treatment of a variety of thoracolumbar injuries using a posterior approach requires a thorough understanding of the mechanism of injury, the integrity of specific structural components of the spine, and the resulting nuances specific to realignment, decompression (if necessary), and instrumentation of each injury type. The posterior approach encompasses a variety of techniques rather than a single method and allows the surgeon to apply specific forces on the spine that are contingent on the exact type of injury. In this chapter, general principles of posterior treatment of thoracolumbar burst fractures, fracture-dislocations, extension injuries, and bending injuries (Chance fractures and flex-ion-distraction injuries) are described. The mechanisms of injury for these fractures have been discussed elsewhere in this monograph; therefore, their brief mention here is simply to provide a context for explaining recommended treatment methods.

BURST FRACTURES

The treatment of burst fractures is perhaps the most justifiably controversial of the fractures discussed in this chapter; specifically, the indications for surgical intervention and the surgical approaches themselves remain debated. The advantages of surgical treatment, even in fractures considered unstable or associated with neurologic deficits, have yet to be reproduced.[1-14] In those who prefer surgical treatment, anterior,[15-22] posterior,[23-26] and combined[27,28] approaches all have strong advocates.

We generally advocate decompression and stabilization of burst fractures with neurologic deficits. In neurologically intact patients, however, the indications are less well defined and highly contingent on individual patient factors. In these patients, the principal indications for surgical stabilization include the following: (1) the presence of a three-column burst fracture in which the posterior column injury is a facet subluxation or equivalent injury rather than the relatively benign nondisplaced vertical lamina fracture;[5,29] (2) the presence of multiple associated injuries; (3) the inability to effectively brace the patient

FIGURE 1

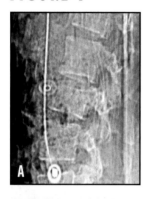
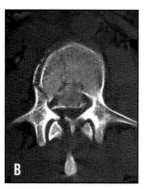
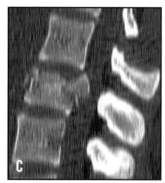
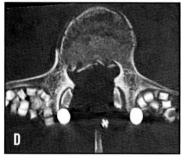
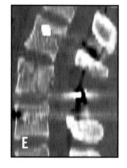
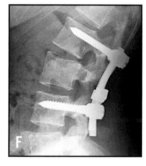

Posterior treatment of an L2 burst fracture with 60% canal compromise in a 24-year-old woman with American Spinal Injury Association (ASIA) D incomplete neurologic injury as a result of a horseback riding accident. **A**, Lateral radiograph. **B**, Preoperative axial CT scan. **C**, Preoperative sagittal CT scan. Postoperative axial **(D)** and sagittal **(E)** CT scans show acceptable spinal canal decompression and vertebral body reconstitution following kyphoreduction, posterior decompression, and reduction of retropulsed fracture fragments via ligamentotaxis and ventral disimpaction. **F**, The alignment remains unchanged 1 year postoperatively with complete motor recovery.

because of other injuries or body habitus; and (4) the anticipated morbidity associated with prolonged periods of recumbency. Kyphosis of 25° or more and loss of more than 50% of vertebral body height are independently considered relative indications.[30]

Benefits of Early Treatment

We believe that early treatment with posterior decompression, kyphoreduction, and short segment instrumentation can be effective, particularly in patients with incomplete spinal cord, conus medullaris, or cauda equina injuries. Early treatment facilitates patient mobilization and nursing care, especially in trauma patients with multiple injuries; offers the best environment for potential recovery of neurologic deficits; and helps restore anatomic spinal alignment and canal patency, either through ligamentotaxis with or without laminectomy or through more direct decompression by ventral disimpaction of retropulsed fracture fragments (Figure 1). Of particular importance in trauma patients with multiple injuries is the expeditious manner in which these goals can be achieved through the posterior approach. In these patients, the posterior approach minimizes the additional physiologic challenges that might result from a thoracotomy and the additional

blood loss with resulting fluid shifts that may be anticipated with a primary anterior or combined approach.[26,31] In the long term, favorable outcomes can also be achieved with a posterior approach, particularly in neurologically intact patients.[24,32]

Realignment and Decompression

Realignment and decompression techniques that use a posterior approach should be familiar to most spine surgeons. We prefer pedicle screw fixation almost universally in the posterior treatment of thoracolumbar injuries because of its unmatched three-column fixation and the versatility it affords in allowing for correction of deformity and in minimizing the number of vertebral levels that require fixation. Our preference is to place the pedicle screws under lateral fluoroscopic guidance once the exposure has been completed, using a consistent starting point throughout the thoracic and lumbar spine at the junction of the transverse process and lateral margin of the corresponding superior facet. Even in patients with extremely narrow thoracic pedicles, we have found that this relatively lateral starting point permits safe placement of screws with lateral penetration along the costovertebral margin posteriorly while allowing excellent anterior purchase within the vertebral body[33] (Figure 2).

In patients with favorable bone quality and screw purchase, fixation is generally limited to the levels directly above and below the burst fracture, particularly in the lumbar spine where preservation of motion segments is more important.[34] The relatively few patients in whom either screw purchase is suboptimal or potential second-stage anterior reconstruction would be prohibitive are treated with longer posterior constructs extending at least two levels rostral and caudal to the injury. In patients with neurologic deficits or in neurologically intact patients with a worrisome degree of canal compromise, a laminectomy is subsequently performed with a high-speed burr and curets using a bilateral trough technique, which eliminates the need for placing bulky rongeurs within a narrowed spinal canal during decompression. Given the more caudal position of the laminae to their corresponding vertebral body, the inferior half of the lamina belonging to the vertebra above the injury level must also be removed to decompress the canal at the level of the retropulsed bony fragments, which tend to occur adjacent to the superior end plate of the injured vertebra (Figure 1, E).

Traumatic dural tears are treated using standard techniques.[35,36] Kyphoreduction is performed by contouring rods into the appropriate amount of lordosis and securing them initially to the cephalad screws. Because of the relative kyphosis at the injured level, the caudal aspect of the rods, once secured to the cephalad screws, lies posterior to the caudal screws before reduction. In translating the caudal end of the rods anteriorly to engage the corresponding caudal screws, the facet joint at the injured level serves as a fulcrum that facilitates correction of kyphosis, as shown in the postoperative CT scans in Figure 1. This correction of alignment, in conjunction with the ligamentotaxis effect of gentle distraction, generally results in considerable canal decompression.[37-40] Any distraction, however, should be undertaken with caution, particularly in neurologically intact patients in whom the risks of distraction may exceed potential benefits.[41,42] Ligamentotaxis alone is less likely to be effective in patients being treated on a more delayed basis (> 24 hours) or in patients with either severe fracture displacement or in whom retropulsed fragments are completely malrotated.[43,44] In these latter two situations, the integrity of the posterior longitudinal ligament and any remaining anular attachment to the retropulsed fragments, upon which the ligamentotaxis effect is largely dependent,[45] are likely to be compromised. AP radiographs assist in determining

FIGURE 2

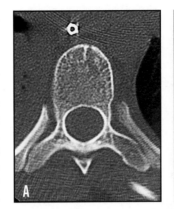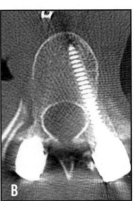

Preoperative **(A)** and postoperative **(B)** axial CT scans through T8 demonstrate safe insertion of pedicle screws with a partially lateral extrapedicular course, which still permits vertebral body purchase. The contralateral screw is viewed on more caudal slices.

the need for preferential distraction of a specific side to correct any coronal-plane malalignment.

Following indirect reduction and stabilization, the extent of residual anterior compression can be assessed by passing a curved instrument along the medial pedicle of the fractured vertebra, just lateral to the traversing nerve root and anterior to the dural sac. Persistent dorsal bulging of the dura and absence of dural pulsations also suggest continued canal compromise. In neurologically compromised patients, any perceived residual canal compromise is addressed by pushing remaining retropulsed fragments anteriorly into the vertebral body and intervertebral space using either a down-biting curet or narrow, angled (footed) impactor. In these situations, the instrument must be passed anterior to the traversing nerve root, taking care to avoid retraction of the neural elements, particularly at the conus medullaris and spinal cord levels. This goal can be facilitated by removing part of the corresponding pedicle or facet joint.[46-49] However, the lateral displacement of the pedicle in burst fractures often renders these additional measures unnecessary in safely accessing the retropulsed fragments for disimpaction.

In our experience, acceptable spinal alignment and canal decompression can be achieved in most cases with the initial, relatively straightforward posterior procedure. This allows for immediate patient mobilization, even in patients in whom anterior and middle column compromise is of sufficient severity to warrant a second-stage anterior corpectomy and reconstruction.

FIGURE 3

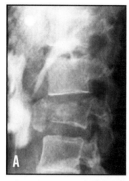
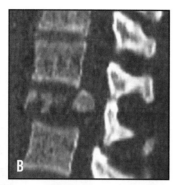
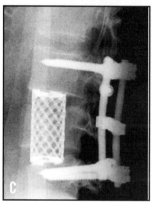
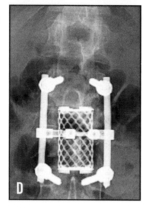

Second-stage anterior surgery after posterior fixation of thoracolumbar burst fracture. Lateral radiograph **(A)** and sagittal CT scan **(B)** of a 36-year-old man who sustained an L2 burst fracture with incomplete ASIA C neurologic injury, a segmental femur fracture, closed head injury, and flail chest as a result of a paragliding accident. He underwent emergent posterior decompression and short segment fixation. Because of the degree of comminution and resultant bony defect, he was subsequently treated with second-stage corpectomy and interbody fusion 1 week postoperatively, as seen in the lateral **(C)** and AP **(D)** radiographs. Early posterior stabilization and decompression eliminated the urgency of performing the more potentially morbid anterior decompression and reconstruction in this patient who sustained injuries to multiple systems and allowed mobilization between procedures.

Factors Influencing the Need for Second-stage Anterior Surgery

The potential need for second-stage anterior surgery is evaluated with postoperative fine-cut CT, which evaluates (1) the adequacy of the decompression in patients with neurologic deficits and (2) the degree of anterior and middle column reconstitution. If either of these elements is found to be unacceptable, second-stage anterior corpectomy and interbody reconstruction can be performed on a semi-elective basis, generally through a limited incision because the presence of posterior instrumentation alleviates the need for supplemental anterior plating. A valid concern with posterior fixation of burst fractures is that, because of the severe vertebral body comminution that is the hallmark of these injuries (Figure 3), unlike with Chance fractures and most flexion-distraction injuries and fracture-dislocations, the anterior and middle columns cannot reasonably contribute to immediate postoperative stability.[50] Anterior compressive forces must therefore be completely absorbed by posterior instrumentation that is suboptimally positioned, from a biomechanical standpoint, to withstand anterior compressive forces.[51] A "race" therefore exists for the vertebral body to consolidate and gradually permit the anterior and middle columns to counteract compressive forces, thus unloading the posterior instrumentation before the fixation fails.

The need for second-stage anterior surgery remains a highly subjective matter. With regard to quantifying the degree of vertebral body integrity as a means of predicting the need for anterior vertebral reconstruction, several authors have suggested general guidelines that may be helpful.[52,53] The rationale is that the greater the degree of comminution and the larger the bony defect, the longer the delay before the posterior instrumentation becomes unloaded, and therefore the higher risk of failure. With regard to the adequacy of decompression, clearly the patient's neurologic status is of key importance, with little tolerance for less than complete decompression in patients with incomplete neurologic deficits.[54,55]

Consistent with the concerns cited above, several authors have described the problem of kyphotic collapse in patients treated with posterior fixation alone.[4,56-58] In our experience, with proper initial restoration of spinal alignment (ie, avoiding initial postoperative kyphosis) and correct screw positioning in nonosteoporotic patients, clinically relevant progression of kyphosis is infrequent.[59] However, it does indeed occur, and reconstruction of patients with late kyphotic collapse is considerably more complex than initial fracture treatment (Figure 4).

FRACTURE-DISLOCATIONS

Fracture-dislocations constitute highly unstable three-column injuries resulting, at least in part, from forces applied to the spine in the transverse plane such as shear and rotation.[60] Although unusual, true facet dislocations may also occur in the thoracolumbar spine. The more

FIGURE 4

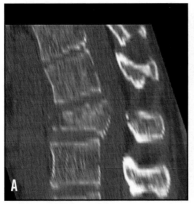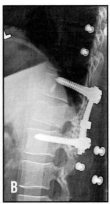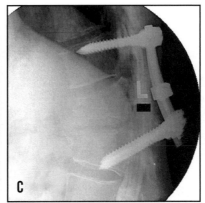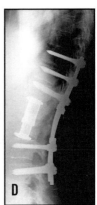

Failure of posterior fixation for thoracolumbar burst fracture. **A,** Lateral radiograph of a 31-year-old patient who sustained a T12 burst fracture with ASIA C incomplete neurologic injury as a result of a motor vehicle accident. **B,** Postoperative lateral radiograph shows restoration of sagittal alignment. **C,** Radiograph obtained 5 months postoperatively reveals failure of fixation with kyphotic collapse, which is a potential risk of posterior burst fracture fixation; in addition, the patient reported increasing pain at this time. **D,** The patient required T12 and L1 corpectomies through a posterolateral (costotransversectomy) approach with simultaneous T9 to L3 posterior arthrodesis and instrumentation.

common pattern involves fracture through the facets or pars interarticularis, with translation and/or rotation about the axial plane (Figure 5). Canal compromise in these injuries is caused primarily by translational/rotational displacement rather than specifically by vertebral body comminution with bony retropulsion, although a combination of these factors may coexist.

Surgical Stabilization

As a general rule, surgical stabilization is recommended for these highly unstable injury patterns, regardless of the patient's neurologic status. We advocate a posterior approach to these injuries for several reasons. (1) Given the highly unstable nature of these injuries, multilevel instrumentation is generally required and cannot be reasonably achieved through a typical anterior approach (Figure 6). (2) Displacement in multiple planes is far more easily correctible through the more versatile and extensile posterior approach than through an anterior exposure. This is more true in patients with actual facet dislocations without associated posterior fracture, where the ability to achieve a reduction without direct visualization of the dislocated facet joints is unlikely. (3) Accurate realignment and stable fixation of these injuries often results in decompression of the spinal canal, even in patients with associated vertebral body fractures.

Most fracture-dislocations present with anterolisthesis, kyphosis, and varying degrees of rotation and lateral lis-

thesis (Figure 5). Kyphosis can be corrected by appropriate lordotic contouring of the rods, as described for kyphoreduction of burst fractures. Anterolisthesis may be simultaneously corrected by positioning the pedicle screw heads cephalad to the injury more anteriorly than those caudal to the injury. As we favor a side-loading pedicle screw system, coronal plane translation and rotation are corrected by sequential approximation of pedicle screws to the rod, initially on the convex side of the deformity, in a manner similar to that described for correction of nontraumatic scoliotic deformities using the so-called translational technique.[61]

The extent of decompression can be enhanced, when considered necessary, by laminectomy. In patients where concerns about potential compression of the neural elements by anterior bony fragments persist, ventral disimpaction of retropulsed fragments may be performed as described for the posterior treatment of unstable burst fractures.[46-49]

Factors Influencing the Need for Second-stage Anterior Surgery

Postoperative CT is useful in determining the need for a second-stage anterior corpectomy and reconstruction. The decision to proceed with subsequent anterior surgery is based on an algorithm similar to that described in the treatment of unstable burst fractures.[52,53] In most cases, any such anterior procedure can be done on a semi-elec-

FIGURE 5

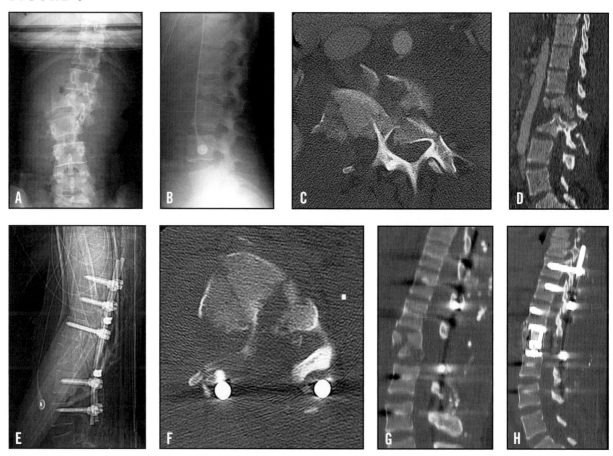

Staged treatment of a thoracolumbar fracture-dislocation. Preoperative AP **(A)** and lateral **(B)** radiographs and axial **(C)** and sagittal **(D)** CT scans of a 26-year-old who sustained multiple traumatic injuries, including an L1-L2 fracture-dislocation with associated L1 ASIA D neurologic deficit, as a result of a motor vehicle accident. Initial treatment with a posterior approach **(E)** was followed by a second-stage anterior corpectomy and interbody reconstruction 2 days later, primarily due to severe vertebral body comminution **(F)** in the presence of mild residual canal compromise **(G)**. Postoperative sagittal CT **(H)** obtained following the second procedure.

tive basis with interim unrestricted patient mobilization, greatly facilitating care of patients with multiple injuries. As with burst fractures, unacceptable residual anterior canal compromise in a neurologically impaired patient is considered grounds for an expeditious approach to the second-stage anterior procedure.[54]

Extension Injuries

Extension injuries, also known as extension-distraction fracture-dislocations, constitute an important subtype of fracture-dislocation.[62] These highly unstable three-column injuries frequently occur in patients with spinal ankylosis due to inflammatory diseases (Figure 7), DISH, or an advanced osteoarthritic process.[63] Thus, these patients are often severely osteoporotic with premorbid kyphotic deformities, both of which are important considerations in their treatment. These injuries are considered high risk given the severe degree of instability and the advanced age and many comorbidities with which patients frequently present.

Because of the extent of instability, we advocate surgical stabilization of these injuries. As a cautionary note, however, standard prone positioning on tables designed to correct more typical kyphosis and anterolisthesis deformities is not recommended because it may actually accentuate these patients' hyperlordosis and retrolisthesis. Consideration should therefore be given to using

FIGURE 6

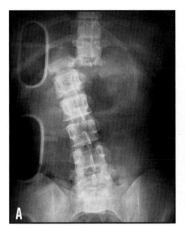
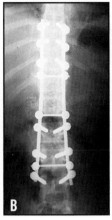
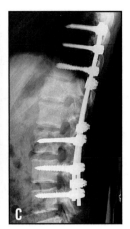

Treatment of a thoracolumbar fracture-dislocation through a posterior approach only. **A,** AP radiograph shows a highly displaced T11-T12 fracture-dislocation with associated fractures of both the T11 and T12 vertebral bodies in a 29-year-old man with ASIA A spinal cord injury, with cord transection, sustained when he fell from his motorcycle and was run over by a truck. Realignment and stabilization of such highly displaced injuries cannot be achieved through anterior surgery and requires a multisegmental posterior exposure. AP **(B)** and lateral **(C)** radiographs obtained 12 months postoperatively show that his alignment remains stable.

alternate positioning techniques, as shown in Figure 7, *D*. The goal should be to restore the patients' premorbid alignment rather than to correct preinjury kyphosis.

The posterior approach is favored in these patients for various reasons, even with the knowledge that posterior fixation violates the mechanical principle of instrumenting the tension side of an injury. First, these injuries may present with severe malalignment, which is far more easily corrected through a posterior multiple-level exposure. Second, the severe osteoporosis commonly seen in these often metabolically compromised patients renders attempts to achieve meaningful fixation through shorter segment anterior instrumentation fruitless and mandates the use of multiple-level three-column instrumentation, and therefore a posterior approach. Correction of residual retrolisthesis can be achieved by positioning the cephalad pedicle screw heads more posterior than those caudal to the injury. Correction of any remaining extension deformity can be achieved by introducing relative kyphosis into the rods and securing them loosely to the pedicle screws at an angle 90° from their intended orientation before finally rotating the rods into their appropriate position, thus correcting the distraction of the anterior spine (Figure 8). Associated coronal plane deformities are corrected in a manner similar to that described for the more typical fracture-dislocations.

FLEXION-DISTRACTION INJURIES AND CHANCE FRACTURES

Because flexion-distraction and Chance fractures result from similar mechanisms that cause the posterior ele-

ments to fail in tension, they are frequently categorized as equivalent "bending" injuries.[64] However, these are distinct injury types, and important nuances between them play an integral role in determining the most favorable approach for posterior stabilization.[65]

Chance Fractures and Their Variants

Chance fractures and their variants are injuries with tension failure that extends from the posterior elements to involve either the vertebral body or intervertebral disk anteriorly, which also fails in tension.[66-68] The axis of rotation is therefore anterior to the vertebral body. Bony Chance fractures may be treated with closed manipulation and a hyperextension cast in neurologically intact patients who do not have associated abdominal and thoracic injuries.

Injuries in adults that compromise the posterior ligaments or intervertebral disk require surgical stabilization. Because these injuries represent a failure in tension of all three spinal columns, vertebral body comminution or bony retropulsion typically is not present. A short segment posterior compression construct therefore provides a force directly antagonistic to the injury force and offers the best mechanical advantage for stabilization of these injuries. A redundant, torn, and/or infolded ligamentum flavum is generally excised before reduction to prevent posterior canal compromise after reduction. Initial reduction can be obtained with interspinous wiring before placement of pedicle screw instrumentation. When the middle column injury involves the posterior anulus, MRI is useful in identifying associated disk herniation that may require excision to minimize the potential

FIGURE 7

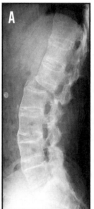
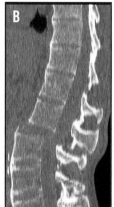
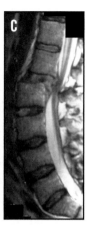

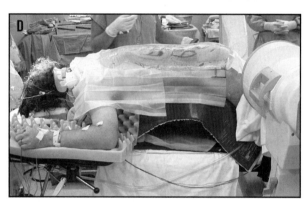

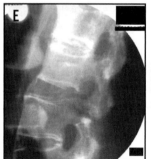
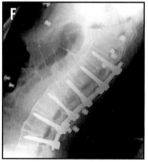

Extension injury treated with a posterior approach. Lateral radiograph (**A**) and sagittal CT scan (**B**) of L1-L2 extension injury resulting from a motor vehicle accident in a 40-year-old man with Behcet's disease and associated spinal ankylosis. Despite the severe canal compromise noted on MRI scan (**C**), the patient remained neurologically intact. Because of concerns that standard prone positioning with a Jackson table (Orthopaedic Systems, Inc, Union City, CA) could cause additional conus medullaris compression by creating additional lordosis and/or retrolisthesis at the fracture site, a Wilson frame (Orthopaedic Systems, Inc) was used (**D**), resulting in improved alignment (**E**). Uneventful posterior decompression, reduction, and stabilization ensued (**F**).

FIGURE 8

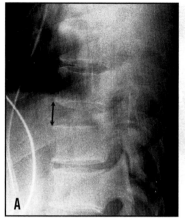
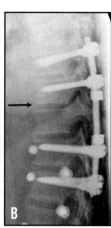

Reduction of an extension injury with a posterior approach. A 43-year-old man who sustained a T9-T10 extension injury in a motor vehicle accident was neurologically intact. After positioning the patient on the operating table, retrolisthesis and anterior distraction persisted (**A**, double arrow). Contouring the rods into relative kyphosis allowed for correction of the deformity (**B**, arrow).

for neurologic injury at the time of posterior compression.[69] Although single-level pedicle screws rostrally and caudally are generally sufficient, the minimum number of levels that need to be spanned depends specifically on the pattern of injury.

If the posterior fracture compromises the pedicles to the extent that solid transpedicular fixation cannot be reliably achieved, extending the stabilization construct to a higher vertebral level is warranted. We have found, however, that in many patients with favorable bone quality in which the posterior fracture involves only the inferiormost aspect of the pedicles, acceptable pedicle screw fixation can be achieved without the need to extend fixation to more rostral levels.

If the fracture extends through bone in all three spinal columns and the posterior column fracture allows for acceptable pedicle screw fixation, then direct repair of the fracture is possible by compressing between the pedicle screws above the fracture and the sublaminar hooks below the fracture, thereby avoiding the need for fusion of any intervertebral level (Figure 9). Extension of the middle and/or anterior column components through the intervertebral disk space requires that at least the vertebrae above and below the disk injury be spanned by the fixation, regardless of the posterior fracture pattern.

FIGURE 9

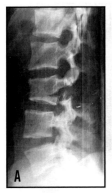
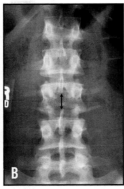
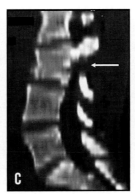
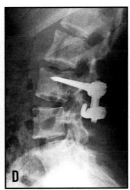
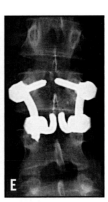

Preoperative lateral **(A)** and AP **(B)** radiographs of a neurologically intact 14-year-old girl with multiple injuries, including a bony Chance fracture and associated abdominal viscus rupture requiring laparotomy. Since the fracture involved only the inferior pedicle cortex **(C**, arrow), direct repair with posterior pedicle screw and hook compression instrumentation was performed. Lateral **(D)** and AP **(E)** radiographs obtained 18 months postoperatively show that the alignment remains stable.

Flexion-Distraction Injuries

There are important distinctions between flexion-distraction injuries and Chance fractures that prove useful in identifying and managing these injuries.[70,71] The flexion-distraction injury, in the strictest sense, is an injury in which the posterior column fails in tension, but, unlike with the Chance fracture, the anterior column fails in compression (Figure 10). The posterior vertebral cortex normally remains intact or fails in tension.[65,70,72] The axis of rotation in these injuries is presumably within the vertebral body rather than in the more anterior location ascribed to Chance fractures. This distinction is important for two reasons: (1) When the tension failure of the posterior elements is unrecognized, these injuries may be incorrectly treated as simple compression fractures based on the frequently more obvious bony injury. Attempts to simply brace these injuries are likely to result in continued kyphotic collapse and the eventual need for a more complex late reconstruction. (2) The preserved integrity or simple tension failure of the posterior vertebral cortex allows it to act as a fulcrum, making the same short segment posterior compression construct used with Chance fractures biomechanically ideal for the treatment of these injuries. This goal can be accomplished either with bisegmental fixation that bypasses the fractured vertebral body or with monosegmental fixation in patients with acceptable bone quality (Figure 10), applying the same caveat as in Chance fractures with regard to possible associated disk herniation.[69,72]

Variants of these fractures do exist in which, despite an injury pattern most consistent with a flexion-distraction mechanism, the injury departs from the classic presentation in that there is comminution of the middle column that extends into the posterior vertebral cortex, suggesting an axial loading (burst) component (Figure 11). Because of the pattern of middle column compromise, these injuries are often described as burst fracture variants.[73] Since the flexion-distraction instability pattern predominates, it is important that these injuries not be treated as standard three-column burst fractures because (1) in our experience they respond less well to nonsurgical treatment, which results in progressive kyphosis, and (2) they are less amenable to anterior fixation than are burst fractures, because instead of neutralizing what would be a burst fracture's primarily axial compressive forces from a mechanically advantageous interbody position, the fixation must counteract rotational forces from a mechanically disadvantageous position near their center of rotation (Figure 12).

This possible presence of middle column comminution also distinguishes flexion-distraction injuries from Chance-type fractures, where tension failure of the middle column is the rule. This possibility presents an important caveat to the universal use of posterior compression instrumentation for treating these injuries. In this latter flexion-distraction variant, the bony elements of the middle column cannot be used as a fulcrum for posterior compression instrumentation without the risk of shortening the middle column and causing bony retropulsion. In flexion-distraction injuries in which there is com-

FIGURE 10

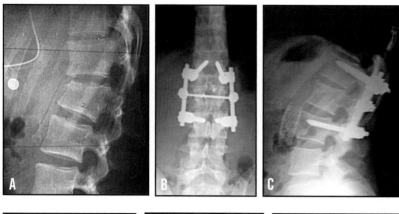

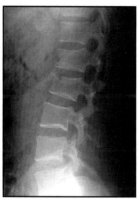
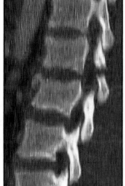
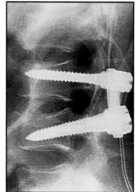

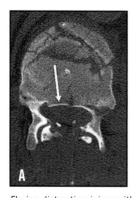
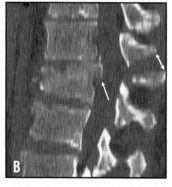

A 21-year-old man sustained an L1-L2 flexion-distraction injury (**A**) and associated aortic injury and duodenal rupture in a motor vehicle accident in which he was the driver and wearing a seat belt. He was neurologically intact. After placement of an aortic stent and laparotomy with bowel repair, L1-L3 posterior compression fixation was performed; the patient had stable alignment 3 years postoperatively (**B and C**). Alternatively, monosegmental fixation also may be used in patients with acceptable bone quality, by directing the pedicle screws toward the inferior end plate of the fractured vertebra (**D, E, and F**).

FIGURE 11

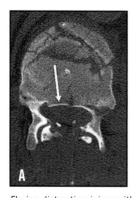

Flexion-distraction injury with middle column comminution. Axial (**A**) and sagittal (**B**) CT scans show middle column fracture and bony retropulsion (single arrow) in this otherwise typical flexion-distraction injury with tension failure through the posterior elements (double arrow) and compression failure of the anterior column. Because of the middle column comminution, posterior compression should not be applied when instrumenting. These injuries should not be misinterpreted as typical three-column burst fractures.

minution that extends into the posterior vertebral cortex, kyphoreduction must instead be achieved without shortening the middle column in a manner similar to that described for posterior stabilization of unstable burst fractures.[74] In this situation, any distraction must be applied with caution since the prevailing tension failure of the posterior elements can lead to overdistraction and neurologic injury and/or kyphosis.

POSTOPERATIVE BRACING

Although the benefits and necessity of postoperative bracing are unconfirmed, we generally prescribe a thoracolumbosacral orthosis (TLSO) (CTLSO for injuries above T7 and HTLSO for injuries below L3), when feasible, to provide supplemental support for 3 months after surgery. The decision to use a postoperative brace, however, depends on patient factors. The information provided here merely constitutes a general protocol. Postoperative bracing is not routinely used in the follow-

FIGURE 12

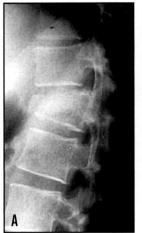 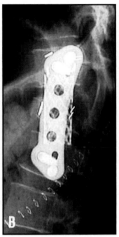 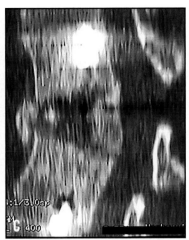 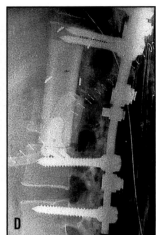

Failure of the anterior approach for treatment of flexion-distraction injury **(A)** in a neurologically intact patient. This approach to stabilizing flexion-distraction injuries makes correction of kyphosis difficult as demonstrated by persistent kyphosis on the postoperative lateral radiograph **(B)**. It also results in suboptimal stability as a result of the biomechanically disadvantaged position of the fixation construct near the center of sagittal plane rotation, which increases the potential for late kyphotic collapse **(C)**. A three-stage anterior and posterior reconstruction was required **(D)**.

ing patients: (1) those with acceptable bone quality who had injury patterns (Chance fractures, flexion-distraction injuries with intact posterior vertebral cortex) amenable to straightforward posterior compression instrumentation; (2) those who have undergone anterior and posterior surgery; (3) those who have a body habitus or associated injuries that preclude effective bracing; or (4) those who are extremely frail or unable to tolerate a brace because of associated pulmonary or skin conditions. Patients are generally mobilized to the same extent postoperatively, regardless of the ability to brace them, with immediate construct stability confirmed by standing radiographs.

CONCLUSION

The posterior approach offers an extensile and straightforward means for effectively stabilizing most thoracolumbar spine injuries while simultaneously allowing sufficient anterior access to effectively decompress the anterior spinal canal. Although not specifically discussed because they are rarely used in the acute treatment of thoracolumbar fractures, the versatility of standard posterior methods may be further enhanced with posterolateral techniques that allow wider visualization and reconstruction of the anterior and middle columns[75] (Figure 4). With the application of three-column posterior fixation techniques throughout the thoracic and lumbar spines,

most thoracolumbar fractures can be effectively treated through the relatively facile and multipurpose posterior approach.

REFERENCES

1. Wood K, Butterman G, Mehbod A, et al: Operative compared with nonoperative treatment of a thoracolumbar burst fracture without neurological deficit: A prospective, randomized study. *J Bone Joint Surg Am* 2003;85:773-781.

2. Chakera TM, Bedbrook G, Bradley CM: Spontaneous resolution of spinal canal deformity after burst-dispersion fracture. *AJNR Am J Neuroradiol* 1988;9:779-785.

3. Boerger TO, Limb D, Dickson RA: Does 'canal clearance' affect neurologic outcome after thoracolumbar burst fractures? *J Bone Joint Surg Br* 2000;82:629-635.

4. Shen WJ, Liu TJ, Shen YS: Nonoperative treatment versus posterior fixation for thoracolumbar junction burst fractures without neurologic deficit. *Spine* 2001;26:1038-1045.

5. Shen WJ, Shen YS: Nonsurgical treatment of three-column thoracolumbar junction burst fractures without neurologic deficit. *Spine* 1999;24:412-415.

6. de Klerk LW, Fontijne WP, Stijnen T, et al: Spontaneous remodeling of the spinal canal after conservative management of thoracolumbar burst fractures. *Spine* 1998;23:1057-1060.

7. Chow GH, Nelson BJ, Gebhard JS, et al: Functional outcome of thoracolumbar burst fractures managed with hyperextension casting or bracing and early mobilization. *Spine* 1996;21:2170-2175.

8. Hitchon PW, Torner JC, Haddad SF, Follett KA: Management options in thoracolumbar burst fractures. *Surg Neurol* 1998;49:619-627.

9. Kraemer WJ, Schemitsch EH, Lever J, et al: Functional outcome of thoracolumbar burst fractures without neurological deficit. *J Orthop Trauma* 1996;10:541-544.

10. Limb D, Shaw DL, Dickson RA: Neurological injury in thoracolumbar burst fractures. *J Bone Joint Surg Br* 1995;77:774-777.

11. Weinstein JN, Collalto P, Lehmann TR: Thoracolumbar "burst" fractures treated conservatively: A long-term follow-up. *Spine* 1988;13:33-38.

12. McEvoy RD, Bradford DS: The management of burst fractures of the thoracic and lumbar spine: Experience in 53 patients. *Spine* 1985;10:631-637.

13. Dickson JH, Harrington PR, Erwin WD: Results of reduction and stabilization of the severely fractured thoracic and lumbar spine. *J Bone Joint Surg Am* 1978;60:799-805.

14. Davies WE, Morris JH, Hill V: An analysis of conservative (non-surgical) management of thoracolumbar fractures and fracture-dislocations with neural damage. *J Bone Joint Surg Am* 1980;62:1324-1328.

15. Ghanayem AJ, Zdeblick TA: Anterior instrumentation in the management of thoracolumbar burst fractures. *Clin Orthop* 1997;335:89-100.

16. Kaneda K, Taneichi H, Abumi K, et al: Anterior decompression and stabilization with the Kaneda device for thoracolumbar burst fractures associated with neurological deficits. *J Bone Joint Surg Am* 1997;79:69-83.

17. Carl AL, Tranmer BI, Sachs BL: Anterolateral dynamized instrumentation and fusion for unstable thoracolumbar and lumbar burst fractures. *Spine* 1997;22:686-690.

18. Okuyama K, Abe E, Chiba M, et al: Outcome of anterior decompression and stabilization for thoracolumbar unstable burst fractures in the absence of neurologic deficits. *Spine* 1996;21:620-625.

19. Shono Y, McAfee PC, Cunningham BW: Experimental study of thoracolumbar burst fractures: A radiographic and biomechanical analysis of anterior and posterior instrumentation systems. *Spine* 1994;19:1711-1722.

20. Gurwitz GS, Dawson JM, McNamara MJ, et al: Biomechanical analysis of three surgical approaches for lumbar burst fractures using short-segment instrumentation. *Spine* 1993;18:977-982.

21. Kostuik JP: Anterior fixation for burst fractures of the thoracic and lumbar spine with or without neurological involvement. *Spine* 1988;13:286-293.

22. McAfee PC, Bohlman HH, Yuan HA: Anterior decompression of traumatic thoracolumbar fractures with incomplete neurological deficit using a retroperitoneal approach. *J Bone Joint Surg Am* 1985;67:89-104.

23. McAfee PC, Yuan HA, Lasda NA: The unstable burst fracture. *Spine* 1982;7:365-373.

24. Leferink VJ, Keizer HJ, Oosterhus JK, et al: Functional outcome in patients with thoracolumbar burst fractures treated with dorsal instrumentation and transpedicular cancellous bone grafting. *Eur Spine J* 2003;12:261-267.

25. Sanderson PL, Fraser RD, Hall DJ, et al: Short segment fixation of thoracolumbar burst fractures without fusion. *Eur Spine J* 1999;8:495-500.

26. Been HD, Bouma GJ: Comparison of two types of surgery for thoraco-lumbar burst fractures: Combined anterior and posterior stabilisation vs. posterior instrumentation only. *Acta Neurochir (Wien)* 1999;141:349-357.

27. Dimar JR II, Wilde PH, Glassman SD, et al: Thoracolumbar burst fractures treated with combined anterior and posterior surgery. *Am J Orthop* 1996;25:159-165.

28. Farcy JP, Weidenbaum M, Glassman SD: Sagittal index in management of thoracolumbar burst fractures. *Spine* 1990;15:958-965.

29. James KS, Wenger KH, Schlegel JD, et al: Biomechanical evaluation of the stability of thoracolumbar burst fractures. *Spine* 1994;19:1731-1740.

30. Willen J, Anderson J, Tomoka K, et al: The natural history of burst fractures at the thoracolumbar junction. *J Spinal Disord* 1990;3:39-46.

31. Danisa OA, Shaffrey CI, Jane JA, et al: Surgical approaches for the correction of unstable thoracolumbar burst fractures: A retrospective analysis of treatment outcomes. *J Neurosurg* 1995;83:977-983.

32. Boucher M, Bhandari M, Kwok D: Health-related quality of life after short segment instrumentation of lumbar burst fractures. *J Spinal Disord* 2001;14:417-426.

33. Dvorak M, MacDonald S, Gurr KR, et al: An anatomic, radiographic, and biomechanical assessment of extra-pedicular screw fixation in the thoracic spine. *Spine* 1993;18:1689-1694.

34. McNamara MJ, Stephens GC, Spengler DM: Transpedicular short-segment fusions for treatment of lumbar burst fractures. *J Spinal Disord* 1992;5:183-187.

35. Denis F, Burkus JK: Diagnosis and treatment of cauda equina entrapment in the vertical lamina fracture of lumbar burst fractures. *Spine* 1991;16(suppl 8):S433-S439.

36. Cammisa FP Jr, Eismont FJ, Green BA: Dural laceration occurring with burst fractures and associated laminar fractures. *J Bone Joint Surg Am* 1989;71:1044-1052.

37. Cain JE Jr, DeJong JT, Dinenber AS, et al: Pathomechanical analysis of thoracolumbar burst fracture reduction: A calf spine model. *Spine* 1993;18:1647-1654.

38. Zou D, Yoo Ju, Edward WT, et al: Mechanics of anatomic reduction of thoracolumbar burst fractures: Comparison of distraction versus distraction plus lordosis, in the anatomic reduction of the thoracolumbar burst fracture. *Spine* 1993;18:195-203.

39. Oda T, Panjabi MM, Kato Y: The effects of pedicle screw adjustments on the anatomical reduction of thoracolumbar burst fractures. *Eur Spine J* 2001;10:505-511.

40. Sjostrom L, Karlstrom G, Pech P, et al: Indirect spinal canal decompression in burst fractures treated with pedicle screw instrumentation. *Spine* 1996;21:113-123.

41. Fidler MW: Remodelling of the spinal canal after burst fracture: A prospective study of two cases. *J Bone Joint Surg Br* 1988;70:730-732.

42. Leferink VJ, Nijboer JM, Zimmerman KW, et al: Burst fractures of the thoracolumbar spine: Changes of the spinal canal during operative treatment and follow-up. *Eur Spine J* 2003;12:255-260.

43. Yazici M, Gulman B, Sen S, Tilki K: Sagittal contour restoration and canal clearance in burst fractures of the thoracolumbar junction (T12-L1): The efficacy of timing of the surgery. *J Orthop Trauma* 1995;9:491-498.

44. Edwards CC, Levine AM: Early rod-sleeve stabilization of the injured thoracic and lumbar spine. *Orthop Clin North Am* 1986;17:121-145.

45. Fredrickson BE, Edwards WT, Rauschning W, et al: Vertebral burst fractures: An experimental, morphologic, and radiographic study. *Spine* 1992;17:1012-1021.

46. Hardaker WT Jr, Cook WA Jr, Fredman AH, et al: Bilateral transpedicular decompression and Harrington rod stabilization in the management of severe thoracolumbar burst fractures. *Spine* 1992;17:162-171.

47. Erickson DLL Jr, Brown WE: One-stage decompression and stabilization for thoracolumbar fractures. *Spine* 1977;2:53-56.

48. Garfin SR, Mowery CA, Guerra J Jr, et al: Confirmation of the posterolateral technique to decompress and fuse thoracolumbar spine burst fractures. *Spine* 1985;10:218-223.

49. Benson DR: Unstable thoracolumbar fractures, with emphasis on the burst fracture. *Clin Orthop* 1988;230:14-29.

50. Panjabi MM, Oxland TR, Lin RM, et al: Thoracolumbar burst fracture. A biomechanical investigation of its multidirectional flexibility. *Spine* 1994;19:578-585.

51. Slosar PJ Jr, Patwardhan AG, Lorenz M, et al: Instability of the lumbar burst fracture and limitations of transpedicular instrumentation. *Spine* 1995;20:1452-1461.

52. McCormack T, Karaikovic E, Gaines RW: The load sharing classification of spine fractures. *Spine* 1994;19:1741-1744.

53. Parker JW, Lane JR, Karaikovic EE, et al: Successful short-segment instrumentation and fusion for thoracolumbar spine fractures: A consecutive 4 1/2-year series. *Spine* 2000;25:1157-1170.

54. Gertzbein SD, Court-Brown CM, Marks P, et al: The neurological outcome following surgery for spinal fractures. *Spine* 1988;13:641-644.

55. Gertzbein SD: Scoliosis Research Society. Multicenter spine fracture study. *Spine* 1992;17:528-540.

56. Alanay A, Acaroglu E, Yazici M, et al: Short-segment pedicle instrumentation of thoracolumbar burst fractures: Does transpedicular intracorporeal grafting prevent early failure? *Spine* 2001;26:213-217.

57. Muller U, Berlemann U, Sledge J, et al: Treatment of thoracolumbar burst fractures without neurologic deficit by indirect reduction and posterior instrumentation: Bisegmental stabilization with monosegmental fusion. *Eur Spine J* 1999;8:284-289.

58. McLain RF, Sparling E, Benson DR: Early failure of short-segment pedicle instrumentation for thoracolumbar fractures: A preliminary report. *J Bone Joint Surg Am* 1993;75:162-167.

59. Yue JJ, Sossan A, Selgrath C, et al: The treatment of unstable thoracic spine fractures with transpedicular screw instrumentation: A 3-year consecutive series. *Spine* 2002;27:2782-2787.

60. McAfee PC, Yuan Ha, Fredrickson BE, et al: The value of computed tomography in thoracolumbar fractures: An analysis of one hundred consecutive cases and a new classification. *J Bone Joint Surg Am* 1983;65:461-473.

61. Aebi MTJ, Thalgott JS, Webb JK (eds): *AO ASIF Principles in Spine Surgery*. New York, Springer-Verlag, 1998.

62. Ferguson RL, Allen BL Jr: A mechanistic classification of thoracolumbar spine fractures. *Clin Orthop* 1984;189:77-88.

63. Hendrix RW, Melany M, Miller F, et al: Fracture of the spine in patients with ankylosis due to diffuse skeletal hyperostosis: Clinical and imaging findings. *AJR Am J Roentgenol* 1994;162:899-904.

64. Denis F: The three column spine and its significance in the classification of acute thoracolumbar spinal injuries. *Spine* 1983;8:817-831.

65. McAfee PC, Yuan HA, Fredrickson BE, Lubicky JP: The value of computed tomography in thoracolumbar fractures: An analysis of one hundred consecutive cases and a new classification. *J Bone Joint Surg Am* 1983;65:461-473.

66. Rogers LF: The roentgenographic appearance of transverse or chance fractures of the spine: The seat belt fracture. *Am J Roentgenol Radium Ther Nucl Med* 1971;111:844-849.

67. Smith WS, Kaufer H: Patterns and mechanisms of lumbar injuries associated with lap seat belts. *J Bone Joint Surg Am* 1969;51:239-254.

68. Chance GQ: Note on a type of flexion fracture of the spine. *Br J Radiol* 1948;21:452.

69. Heller JG, Garfin SR, Abitbol JJ: Disk herniations associated with compression instrumentation of lumbar flexion-distraction injuries. *Clin Orthop* 1992;284:91-98.

70. Gertzbein SD, Court-Brown CM: Flexion-distraction injuries of the lumbar spine: Mechanisms of injury and classification. *Clin Orthop* 1988;227:52-60.

71. Gumley G, Taylor TK, Ryan MD: Distraction fractures of the lumbar spine. *J Bone Joint Surg Br* 1982;64:520-525.

72. Finkelstein JA, Wai EK, Jackson SS, et al: Single-level fixation of flexion distraction injuries. *J Spinal Disord Tech* 2003;16:236-242.

73. Abe E, Sato K, Shimada Y, et al: Thoracolumbar burst fracture with horizontal fracture of the posterior column. *Spine* 1997;22:83-87.

74. Gertzbein SD, Court-Brown CM: Rationale for the management of flexion-distraction injuries of the thoracolumbar spine based on a new classification. *J Spinal Disord* 1989;2:176-183.

75. Larson SJ, Holst RA, Hemmy DC, Sances A Jr: Lateral extracavitary approach to traumatic lesions of the thoracic and lumbar spine. *J Neurosurg* 1976;45:628-637.

CHAPTER 9

EVALUATION AND MANAGEMENT OF THORACOLUMBAR FRACTURES— ANTERIOR APPROACH

KERN SINGH, MD

MATTHEW D. EICHENBAUM, MD

LAURENCE N. FITZHENRY, MD

ALEXANDER R. VACCARO, MD

The thoracolumbar spine is the most common site of vertebral fractures. Most thoracolumbar injuries in the young adult are caused by high-energy trauma such as motor vehicle accidents or falls from a height.[1,2] A multiple-center review of more than 1,000 spinal trauma patients conducted by the Scoliosis Research Society revealed that 16% of injuries occurred between T1 and T10, 52% between T11 and L1, and 32% between L1 and L5.[1-3] Depending on the type of fracture, associated spinal and nonspinal injuries occur in up to 50% of patients.[4] Half of the associated injuries result from a distraction force and may involve injury to intra-abdominal viscera or vessel disruption. Pulmonary injuries occur in approximately 20% of these patients, and intra-abdominal bleeding secondary to liver and splenic injury occurs in about 10%.[5] Contiguous and noncontiguous spinal injuries are present in 6% to 15% of patients.

ANATOMY

Regional thoracic and lumbar anatomic characteristics, the degree and direction of force impact, and a patient's postural alignment all contribute to the degree and pattern of spinal injury. The physiologic kyphosis of the thoracic spine may predispose it to flexion-axial load injuries that may be further aggravated following a surgical laminectomy.[6]

The thoracolumbar junction is a transitional region between the less mobile thoracic spine and the more flexible lumbar spine. This area is referred to as the junctional area and is prone to injury because the rib cage no longer provides protection and support to the vertebral column. Also, the thoracic vertebral bodies are not as large as the lumbar vertebral bodies; thus, they are less able to resist deformity following specific load application. These factors render the thoracolumbar spine more vulnerable to injury and make it the most common location for burst fractures.[4]

IMAGING EVALUATION

The radiographic evaluation of a patient with a suspected thoracolumbar injury begins with AP and lateral radiographs of the entire spine. The lateral view is used to assess alignment of the vertebral bodies, pedicles, facet joints, spinous processes, and intervertebral foramina. The cortical margins of the vertebral bodies should be unbroken so as to form an intact posterior vertebral body line. Disruption of the posterior vertebral body line may signal spinal canal compromise from a burst fracture.[7] Other signs that suggest a compression injury include buckling of the cortical margins, loss of vertebral body height, and an intravertebral vacuum sign. The AP view is used to assess vertebral alignment and vertebral body cortical disruption from a lateral compression fracture that may be missed on the lateral view. Malalignment of midline spinous processes or widening of the interpedicular line may represent significant posterior element injury and instability.

Further clarification of the degree of injury may require CT or MRI. CT is used to evaluate the integrity of the middle column (posterior vertebral body) and the posterior column (posterior elements) of the vertebral body. Approximately 25% of burst fractures may be misdiagnosed as stable compression fractures when viewed on radiographs.[8] MRI has emerged as the definitive diagnostic modality in the evaluation of spinal cord injury.

CLASSIFICATION SYSTEMS

Denis[6] modified and popularized a previous classification system based on a three-column theory of spinal instability. He reviewed 412 patients with thoracic and lumbar fractures and classified the injuries as either major or minor. Minor injuries, which accounted for more than 15% of the fractures, included fractures of the spinous and transverse processes, the pars interarticularis, and the facet articulations. Major injuries were divided into compression fractures, burst fractures, flexion-distraction injuries, and fracture-dislocations.

Ferguson and Allen[9] presented a mechanistic classification of thoracolumbar injuries, describing seven injury patterns (Table 1). This system categorizes injuries by the forces that create them and therefore is useful in guiding nonsurgical and surgical treatment strategies. The seven injury patterns are compressive flexion, distractive flexion, lateral flexion, translational, torsional flexion, vertical compression, and distractive extension injuries.

SURGICAL DECISION MAKING

A popular strategy for addressing the need for surgery is through the assessment of the integrity of the posterior osteoligamentous complex. If findings in a typical burst fracture include marked widening between adjacent spinous processes and obvious kyphotic malalignment, the fracture is considered unstable with the potential for deformity progression. Denis[6] defined instability as a disruption of two or more of the three spinal columns and categorized instability as mechanical, neurologic, or combined. Mechanical instability occurs with fracture patterns involving disruption of multiple columns, specifically of the posterior elements in distraction leading to the potential for late kyphotic deformity. Neurologic instability describes a neurologic

deficit in the setting of a spinal fracture. Combined instability refers to an unstable mechanical fracture along with a neurologic deficit.

The role of spinal decompression as treatment of thoracolumbar injuries with symptomatic neural compression is unclear. Despite varied opinions, radiographic evidence of canal occlusion does not correlate with the severity of neurologic deficit following burst fractures.[10] Rather, the underlying cause of neurologic injury may be a combination of factors, including the initial force on the spinal cord or the cauda equina as well as the associated hematoma, edema, and vascular ischemia caused by various neurotrophic and vasoactive agents.

Anterior Decompression

In selected patients, the anterior approach is preferred over indirect posterior approaches because an anterior approach allows direct visualization of the anterior thecal sac and ensures the potential for optimal neural decompression. Vertebrectomy is often beneficial when used for spinal canal compromise that is the result of retropulsion of vertebral bone and disk fragments in a patient with an incomplete neurologic deficit. Specific fracture patterns are more amenable to an initial anterior approach in patients with incomplete neurologic deficit. For example, an unstable burst fracture or compressive flexion or vertical compression injury with adequate coronal-plane alignment is often approached anteriorly to relieve neural compression and restore stability to the anterior column. Anterior surgery is also beneficial when anterior column support is necessary to prevent late kyphotic collapse and progressive pain. These problems often occur with comminuted, unstable burst fractures (with associated posterior osteoligamentous instability) or flexion compression injuries in neurologically intact patients. Anterior surgery provides significant stability, regardless of the patient's neurologic status, in distractive extension injuries with significant anterior open fishmouth deformities following a posterior stabilization procedure. Anterior column support in this setting may prevent late instability that sometimes occurs if fusion fails to heal.

In patients with significant spinal displacement, such as flexion distraction, fracture-dislocations, or shear injuries, an initial posterior approach is often necessary to restore alignment before anterior thecal sac decompression. After obtaining adequate alignment, the surgeon may then assess the degree of thecal sac impingement by perform-

TABLE 1

Ferguson and Allen Classification System for Spinal Fractures

Type of Fracture	Anterior Column	Middle Column	Posterior Column
Compressive flexion			
Type I	Compression	None	None
Type II	Compression	None	Tension
Type III	Compression	"Hydraulic blowout"*	Tension
Distractive flexion	Tension	Tension	Tension
Lateral flexion			
Type I	Unilateral compression	Unilateral compression	None
Type II	Unilateral compression	Unilateral compression	Ipsilateral compression/contralateral tension
Translational	Shear	Shear	Shear
Torsional flexion	Compression/rotation	Disrupted	Tension/rotation
Vertical compression	Compression	Bony compression	Bony involvement
Distractive extension	Tension		Compression

*Evidence of middle column bone rotated into the neural canal between the pedicles

ing a limited laminoforaminotomy, an intraoperative myelogram, or an intraoperative ultrasound. A posterior anterior approach is also useful when posterior indirect reduction fails to provide adequate neural decompression and a neurologic deficit persists. In approximately 4% of patients with an incomplete neurologic deficit and spinal canal occlusion, persistent neural impingement following posterior reduction may warrant a subsequent posterolateral or anterior decompression.[11] A posterior-anterior procedure also may be used for an open spinal fracture with posterior soft-tissue damage. Following initial posterior débridement, a subsequent anterior stabilization procedure with instrumentation often restores stability.

A circumferential surgical approach may be necessary in certain thoracolumbar injuries. An anterior approach followed by a posterior approach is useful in the stabilization of three-column spinal injuries with significant instability in the setting of symptomatic canal occlusion (Figure 1). If posterior instability persists following anterior decompression and reconstruction, supplemental posterior stabilization is often recommended. This technique is also useful when placement of anterior instru-

mentation may pose a physical risk to the surrounding great vessels because of implant prominence.

A simultaneous combined anterior and posterior spinal approach with the patient in the lateral position may be used for a midthoracic spinal burst-type injury without any coronal-plane deformity. A single-stage simultaneous procedure results in less surgical time and blood loss and fewer complications compared with a two-stage procedure.[12,13]

Biomechanics of the Anterior Approach

Anterior surgery restores the load-bearing function of the anterior spine. Direct access to the anterior vertebral body allows accurate placement of an optimally sized interbody spacer, thereby decreasing the potential for graft displacement and subsequent deformity. It it important to remember that 80% of the axial load transmitted through the spine is through the intact anterior column. Obviously, a thoracolumbar fracture disrupts this physiologic load-bearing capacity. Therefore, during anterior column reconstruction, insertion of the implant in an intracolumnar position allows it to function as an interbody spacer and load-sharing device, restoring axial stability

FIGURE 1

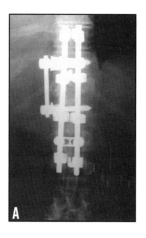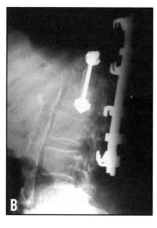

AP **(A)** and lateral **(B)** radiographs following an anterior-posterior stabilization procedure for a fracture-dislocation of the thoracic spine.

until arthrodesis occurs. With a deficient anterior column and no structural interbody spacer, a posterior spinal construct bears most of the axially applied loads, leading to the potential for nonunion of the arthrodesis and early instrumentation failure.

For nonpathologic fractures of the thoracolumbar spine, reconstruction of the anterior spinal column is performed with a biologically active graft to optimize bony incorporation and long-term stability (Figure 2). The most commonly used interbody spacer is an autologous tricortical iliac crest, although allograft sources such as a tibial or femoral shaft or metallic mesh cages are gaining popularity. Recently introduced expandable cages avoid the need to insert the device through a slightly oversized compression fit. The surgeon can "dial" the degree of distraction necessary to restore sagittal plane alignment. This method of reconstruction somewhat conflicts with Wolff's law in that the grafting material within the cage is obviously unloaded during distraction of the expandable cage. To date, fusion healing has not been adversely affected. Long-term outcome studies on these devices have not yet been published.

Iliac crest interbody grafts, compared with allograft strut grafts, allow for a faster rate of bony incorporation given their biocompatibility. However, allograft strut grafts are able to withstand greater physiologic loads in the erect spine in the early reconstruction and healing period.[13] Several authors have reported successful results using anterior cortical allograft strut grafts in thoracolumbar frac-

tures; at 5-year follow-up, fusion rates exceed 90% with minimal graft subsidence and change in sagittal alignment.[14,15] In late posttraumatic kyphosis, nonunion and loss of correction often occur in up to 50% of patients when anterior interbody grafts are used without supplemental internal fixation. In this situation, adjunctive posterior internal fixation is recommended (with or without possible anterior instrumentation) to prevent recurrence of the spinal deformity.

TECHNICAL ASPECTS OF THE ANTERIOR APPROACH

The anterolateral approach to the spine (transthoracic T4 to T9, thoracoabdominal T10 to L1, or retroperitoneal T12 to L5) is the most common way to expose the anterolateral thoracolumbar vertebral bodies. A right-sided approach is commonly used for exposures above T10 because of interference with the heart and associated great vessels. For ease of visualization, the initial exposure and the rib to be resected are at the same level as the injured vertebral body or one to two levels above it. The parietal pleura is exposed and incised halfway between the neuroforamen and the great vessels. Once the vertebral body is identified, a radiograph is obtained to confirm the appropriate spinal level. The segmental vessels over the injured vertebral body are identified and ligated if necessary. The pleura, segmental vessels, and periosteum are elevated with the use of a bovie, key elevator, and peanuts, thereby allowing placement of a blunt Homan retractor between the anterior spine and aorta. A narrow Homan or Penfield 4 retractor is placed within the neuroforamen at the lateral border of the spinal canal to facilitate soft-tissue retraction laterally. The adjacent disks are sharply incised and removed individually with curved curets, rongeurs, and straight pituitaries. Next, the superior and inferior boundaries of the pedicle are identified, followed by removal of the pedicle with a Kerrison punch and cutting burr, if necessary. This step allows the nerve root to be identified and followed to its intersection with the thecal sac. In the thoracic spine, the costovertebral junction articulates with the cephalad portion of its respective vertebral body. Removal of this articulation with a rongeur allows exposure of the underlying pedicle. Once the pedicle has been removed, the posterior boundary of the vertebral body is identified to facilitate removal of the vertebral body. An osteotome is used initially to remove

FIGURE 2

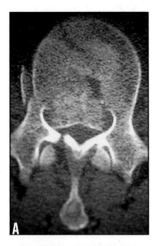
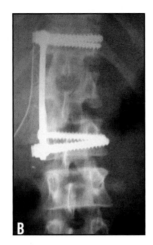

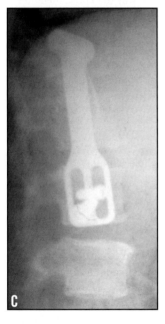

A, Preoperative axial CT scan of a patient who sustained an L1 burst fracture and a neurologically incomplete conus medullaris injury after falling from a ladder. The posterior vertebral body is retropulsed into the spinal canal, with approximately 85% canal narrowing. Postoperative AP **(B)** and lateral **(C)** radiographs following an L1 corpectomy and fusion using an autologous iliac crest strut graft, followed by placement of an anterior plate and screw stabilization.

the anterior two thirds of the vertebral body, leaving a portion of the anterior vertebral body wall to protect against subsequent graft displacement. A burr and curved curets are then used to remove the remaining vertebral body down to the posterior longitudinal ligament. Decompression is continued until the medial border of the contralateral pedicle is identified.

Anterior Instrumentation

With the continued refinement of anterior fixation devices, supplementary posterior fixation and fusion is being performed less frequently in select spinal injuries. Anterior fusion constructs offer the best chance for bony healing when supported by an intact posterior-element tension band. In the absence of significant posterior osteoligamentous disruption, an anterior procedure alone, using a dual rod or plating fixation device, may confer adequate stability and avoid the need for a posterior procedure.[16,17] If significant posterior instability exists, or if more than one vertebral body has been resected, a second-stage posterior stabilization and fusion procedure usually is recommended. An anterior spinal implant may also function as a neutralization device to span a grafted spinal defect in the setting of a planned posterior stabilization procedure. Some older anterior systems were associated with the potential for late injury to the great vessels given their prominence and excessive anterior spinal placement, but newer systems are lower profile and surgeons are more cognizant of the importance for lateral placement along the vertebral body.

Anterior thoracolumbar surgery is a technically demanding procedure that is not without significant potential complications. Oskouian and Johnson[18] retrospectively reviewed 207 patients who underwent anterior thoracolumbar decompression and reconstruction. Vascular complications developed in 12 patients (5.8%), and 2 patients (1%) died. Deep venous thrombosis developed in 5 patients (2.4%), with 1 patient dying from a pulmonary embolism.

SUMMARY AND CONCLUSIONS

The management of thoracolumbar injuries continues to be controversial. Despite advances in anesthesia and implant technology, disagreement still exists over basic issues involving the need for surgery, the timing of surgical intervention, and the appropriate approach for specific fracture patterns. Nonetheless, treatment should be guided by an understanding of spinal anatomy, biomechanics, and by a detailed examination of the specific injury type and overall medical condition of the patient. Although the need and timing of surgical intervention for spinal injury is debated, aggressive medical management with early patient mobilization is beneficial for the overall functional recovery of the patient. Most thoracolumbar injuries, in the absence of a neurologic deficit, are stable and can be successfully treated nonsurgically. For the rare unstable spinal fracture, with or without a neurologic deficit, surgery improves patient mobilization and allows early functional return to society. The ultimate goals in management are to maximize neurologic recovery and to expeditiously stabilize the spine for early rehabilitation and an early return to a productive lifestyle.

REFERENCES

1. Burgos J, Rapariz JM, Gonzalez-Herranz P: Anterior endoscopic approach to the thoracolumbar spine. *Spine* 1998;23:2427-2431.

2. Carpenter MB: *Core Text of Neuroanatomy*, ed 4. Baltimore, MD, Williams & Wilkins, 1991.

3. Kraus JF, Franti CE, Biggin RS, Richards D, Bohrani NO: Incidence of traumatic spinal cord lesions. *J Chronic Dis* 1975;28:471-492.

4. Rizzolo DJ, Piazza MR, Cotler JM: Intervertebral disc injury complicating cervical spine trauma. *Spine* 1991;16:187-189.

5. Dick W, Kluger P, Magerl F: A new device for internal fixation of thoracolumbar and lumbar spine fractures: The "fixateur intern." *Paraplegia* 1985;23:225-232.

6. Denis F: The three column spine and its significance in the classification of acute thoracolumbar spinal injuries. *Spine* 1983;8:817-831.

7. Brown CW, Gorup JM, Chow GH: Nonsurgical treatment of thoracic burst fractures in controversies, in Zdeblick TA, Benzel EC, Anderson PA, Stillerman CB (eds): *Spine Surgery*. St Louis, MO, Quality Medical Publishing, 1999, pp 86-96.

8. Flanders AE: Thoracolumbar trauma imaging overview. *Instr Course Lect* 1999;48:429-431.

9. Ferguson RL, Allen BL Jr: A mechanistic classification of thoracolumbar spine fractures. *Clin Orthop* 1984;189:77-88.

10. Cantor JB, Lebwohl NH, Garvey T, Eismont FJ: Non-operative management of stable thoracolumbar burst fractures with early ambulation and bracing. *Spine* 1993;18:971-976.

11. Edwards WT, Zheng Y, Ferrara LA, Yuan HA: Structural features and thickness of the vertebral cortex in the thoracolumbar spine. *Spine* 2001;26:218-225.

12. Dick JC, Brodke DS, Zdeblick TA, Bartel BD, Kunz DN, Rapoff AJ: Anterior instrumentation of the thoracolumbar spine: A biomechanical comparison. *Spine* 1997;22:744-750.

13. Stancic MF, Gregorovic E, Nozica E, Penezic L: Anterior decompression and fixation versus posterior reposition and semirigid fixation in the treatment of unstable burst thoracolumbar fracture: Prospective clinical trial. *Croat Med J* 2001;42:49-53.

14. Finkelstein JA, Chapman JR, Mirza S: Anterior cortical allograft in thoracolumbar fractures. *J Spinal Disord* 1999;12:424-429.

15. Singh K, Dewald CJ, Hammberberg KW, Dewald RL: Long structural allografts in the treatment of anterior spinal column defects. *Clin Orthop* 2002;394:121-129.

16. Breeze SW, Doherty BJ, Noble PS, LeBlanc A, Heggeness MH: A biomechanical study of anterior thoracolumbar screw fixation. *Spine* 1998;23:1829-1831.

17. Kotani Y, Cunningham BW, Parker LM, Kanayama M, McAfee PC: Static and fatigue biomechanical properties of anterior thoracolumbar instrumentation systems: A synthetic testing model. *Spine* 1999;24:1406-1413.

18. Oskouian RJ, Johnson JP: Vascular complications in anterior thoracolumbar spinal reconstruction. *J Neurosurg* 2002;96(suppl 1):1-5.

CHAPTER 10

GUNSHOT INJURY TO THE THORACOLUMBAR SPINE

RONALD W. LINDSEY, MD
ZBIGNIEW GUGALA, MD, PHD

Gunshot injuries have become extremely prevalent in the United States among the civilian, nonmilitary population due to the increase in gun availability and urban violence.[1-4] Accordingly, there has been a dramatic increase in gunshot injuries to the spine, especially in urban areas where they can comprise 13% of all spinal injuries, ranking third only to falls and motor vehicle accidents.[5,6] There has also been a dramatic increase in the incidence of spinal cord injury as a result of civilian gunshot injuries over the past several decades. Data from the National Spinal Cord Injury Model System Database demonstrated that gunshot injury-related spinal cord injury has almost doubled from 13% to 25% over a 20-year period.[7] Civilian gunshot injuries to the spine in urban regions constitute the second most common cause of all spinal cord injuries following motor vehicle accidents but occurring more frequently than falls.[8-11]

McKinley and associates[10] demonstrated that blunt spinal cord injury patients differ epidemiologically from ballistic spinal cord injury patients, primarily in terms of their ethnicity, socioeconomic status, and injury severity. Typically, ballistic spinal cord injury patients are young males age 25 to 30 years,[4,9,11] 92% of whom are either black or Hispanic.[9,10,12] These patients usually sustain their spine injuries in the thoracic region (50% to 60%), and approximately 80% of these patients experience additional morbidity due to major associated injuries to the lungs, viscera, and major vessels.[8-10,13] In 1998 Eismont[14] estimated the survivability of a gunshot injury, in general, to be 83% due to advances in modern trauma health care. However, when the spine is involved the prognosis is often poor.[15]

BALLISTICS

Ballistics characterizes three phases of projectile motion: its passage through the barrel of a firearm (interior ballistics), subsequent projectile trajectory through the air (external ballistics), and projectile penetration of the target (terminal ballistics). Wound ballistics is a part of the terminal ballistics that characterizes the motion and interactions of a projectile in living tissues.

All firearms can be classified into three major categories according to their muzzle velocity: low-velocity (< 350 m/s), medium-velocity (350 to 600 m/s), and high-velocity (> 600 m/s). Handguns, except for magnums, are low-velocity; shotguns and magnum handguns are medium-velocity; high-velocity weapons are usually rifles. Gunshot wounds in civilians are typically the result of low- or medium-velocity firearms. Muzzle velocity alone does not determine the wounding potential of a firearm, and, therefore, the type of firearm is not synonymous with the type of wound created.[16-18] The type of bullet used can greatly impact wounding, and this is most evident with shotguns. Although shotguns are medium-velocity weapons, the large total mass of their lead pellets dramatically increases their kinetic energy. Depending on the distance to the target and the size of pellets, shotguns can possess the wounding potential of high-velocity firearms or multiple low-velocity weapons.

WOUNDING POTENTIAL

The wounding potential of a projectile reflects its kinematics and physical characteristics after entering the target tissue. The primary determinant of missile wounding potential is the amount of its energy dissipated within the tissue after impact. Missile deceleration and subsequent energy transfer are functions of the missile energy on entry (impact energy), distance to the target missile design, characteristics of the target tissue, and missile behavior within the tissue.[19]

Impact Energy

Total kinetic energy of the missile striking the target is the sum of advancing and rotational missile energy and is proportional to the missile mass and the impact velocity squared ($\sim mv^2$). In general, an impact velocity of approximately 50 m/s is necessary to penetrate the skin, whereas a velocity of 65 m/s is needed to fracture bone.[20] The missile's impact and muzzle energies are not equivalent, because some of the missile energy dissipates during flight. The magnum shell of a firearm enhances the muzzle velocity of the bullet 20% to 60% by increasing the gunpowder charge. High-mass missiles (ie, shotgun pellets) can result in a high-energy injury even if inflicted by a low- or medium-velocity weapon.[21] It is important to appreciate the amount of energy transferred to the tissue, as this energy constitutes the major wounding potential of a missile. The designation of the wounding potential based on the type of firearm or its muzzle velocity alone is unreliable, since most of the civilian gunshot injuries are inflicted with low- or medium-velocity weapons.

Distance to the Target

The distance between a firearm and the target has an enormous impact on the missile wounding potential. Missile muzzle energy decreases significantly if the distance to the target exceeds 45 m for low-velocity firearms, or 90 m for high-velocity firearms. The effect of distance to target is best demonstrated with shotguns, where distance to the target is the basis for classifying shotgun severity.[22,23] In contrast to typical civilian bullets, which are pointed, round shotgun pellets have poor aerodynamic properties and lose their kinetic energy rapidly during flight. At close range (< 5 m),

shotgun pellets act essentially as one mass causing massive tissue destruction. The impact energy of a shotgun fired at this distance is similar to that of high-velocity firearm. Very close proximity of the shotgun to the target (< 2 m) results in not only the pellet projection, but also shell fragments and wadding. Pellets projected at a distance of more than 5 m scatter substantially during flight, and their tissue penetration usually is limited to the deep fascia (5 to 12 m) or superficial skin (> 12 m).[22]

Missile Design

The components of missile design such as its geometry, mass, caliber, material, and presence of a jacket affect missile interactions with the target tissue. Civilian bullets typically are made of lead and have no jacket. They deform easily on impact, and demonstrate decreased tissue penetration as well as the increased likelihood of bullet retention, thereby dissipating more energy within the target tissue. Military bullets have a copper jacket (Hague Convention 1899) that prevents bullet deformation, increases tissue penetration, and decreases likelihood of missile retention, thereby lowering energy transfer to the target tissue. The wounding potential of a shotgun is dependent on a "bolus" blast effect, which can be reduced by pellet spreading. Pellets with a diameter less than 0.14 in, commonly known as birdshot (shot number 3 or smaller), can allow as many as 200 to 700 pellets per shell; whereas only 8 to 100 pellets with larger diameters (shot number 3 or larger), so-called buckshot, can fit inside a shell. The wounding potential of buckshot is greater than birdshot, and can be equivalent to multiple low-caliber handgun wounds.

Physical Properties of Target Tissue

Energy dissipation is directly related to the target tissue density and inversely related to the target tissue elasticity. Missiles striking tissues of low density and high elasticity, such as lungs, result in a small energy dissipation and minor wounding. Organs with very low or no elasticity such as the liver, spleen, blood vessels, and neural structures absorb considerable energy and can be damaged significantly. Fluid-filled organs such as the bladder, heart, great vessels, and bowel can explode because of the pressure waves generated upon missile energy transfer. Dense, nonelastic tissues such as bone are of special concern due to the significant amount of energy that can be dissipated, even with short penetration. Secondary missiles caused by bone and/or bullet fragmentation can further compound local tissue damage.

Missile Behavior Within the Tissue

Persistent minor deviations of the bullet from its trajectory during flight increase the energy released in the target tissue. Dense tissues increase the tumbling and yawing of the bullet and result in greater energy dissipation. Likewise, bullet fragmentation within the tissue increases the energy transfer. For nonfragmenting missiles, a longer wound track is necessary to impart their full wounding potential.

CLINICAL CHARACTERISTICS OF GUNSHOT INJURY

Clinical severity of a gunshot injury is determined by the amount of projectile energy dissipated within the tissue after the impact and by the nature and extent of the involvement of the specific anatomic structures of the body.[24] Primary mechanisms of tissue damage result from the physical consequences of a projectile passing through the tissue, and can include laceration and crushing (permanent cavitation); transient displacement and stretching of the tissue radially outward of the projectile track (temporary cavitation); and shock waves propagated remotely within the tissue. Secondary injuring mechanisms may result from displaced bone fragments, or may occur as a result of the victim's falling after the shot.

Injury Energy

The gunshot wounds are designated into low- or high-energy, depending on the extent of the kinetic energy of a projectile dissipated within tissue. Low-energy wounds are typically caused by guns with nonjacketed bullets that create short tracts through less dense and elastic tissues (skin, adipose tissue, muscle, trabecular bone). This low-energy trauma usually is localized to the missile track and results in local cutting and/or crushing mechanisms. In rare circumstances, an injury created by a high-velocity missile to low-density tissues may be considered as low-energy.

In high-energy transfer gunshot injuries, tissue damage is more significant due to the presence of temporary cavitation. In addition, high-energy missiles can create shock waves that propagate in the target tissue and thereby are capable of inflicting remote injuries. High-mass missiles can result in a high-energy injury, even if inflicted by a low- or medium-velocity weapon such as a shotgun.[21] Designating the energy dissipation within the tissue is done by a thorough clinical assessment of the gunshot wound, since the details of the specific type of firearm and the injury circumstances are rarely available to the clinician.

Anatomic Structure Involvement

In designating the clinical severity of the gunshot injury, apart from the missile energy, it is imperative to determine the involvement of the vital anatomic structures and assess the nature and extent of this damage. In select gunshot injuries, the involvement of vital structures can account for greater clinical severity than could be reflected by the ballistic missile wounding potential. In general patient injuries following gunshots can be divided into two major categories: wounds to the vital structures (central and peripheral neural elements, vessels, and viscera) and wounds to the musculoskeletal tissues. Life-saving interventions should be done immediately for injuries that disrupt the airway, compromise breathing, or involve the circulatory system. Gunshot injuries involving musculoskeletal tissues (bone, muscle, joints, ligaments/tendons) can result in morbidity because of instability, severe functional deficit, infection, or the risk for amputation.

Types of Gunshot Wounds

Gunshots can inflict three basic types of wounds that include nonpenetrating, penetrating, and perforating. Nonpenetrating wounds occur without the missile completely entering the target tissue (grazing or blast injury). The depth and area of tissue involved may vary, but typically the injury is restricted to the superficial soft-tissue layers. Penetrating wounds consist of a missile entrance site but no exit. In this setting, the bullet or its fragments are retained within the tissue and the impact kinetic energy of the missile is dissipated within the tissues entirely. In perforating wounds a missile entrance and exit site are present. Clinical distinctions between the entrance and exit sites without knowing the detailed circumstances of the injury can be extremely difficult and misleading.[25] Identification of the bullet entrance and exit sites may assist in establishing bullet trajectory.

Distinguishing between the penetrating and perforating types of gunshot wounds is critical in determining missile retention in the tissue and reflects the amount of missile energy transferred.[26] Retained bullet fragments warrant surgical excision if they are present intra-articularly (including disk space),[27,28] within the spinal canal,[5] or have traversed bowel.[29] Brass- or copper-jacketed bullets lodged in proximity to central or peripheral neural structures may require surgical removal because of their neurotoxicity.[30,31] The depth of the wound created by the missile also provides a good indication of the energy dissipated within the tissue. Theoretically, the energy transferred in penetrating injuries equals the entire missile impact energy, whereas the transferred energy in perforating gunshot wounds is the difference between the entrance and exit energies. Practically, however, a substantial amount of energy is necessary for complete perforation of the target tissues, and this usually occurs with missiles of high-impact energy. Therefore the perforating gunshot injuries tend to be more severe.

Gunshot Injuries to Bone

Gunshot injuries commonly affect bone, causing fractures. The extent of gunshot injury to bone depends on the missile impact energy and the structural properties of the bone affected. Low-energy gunshot injury to porous, low-density, or cancellous bone can result in a "drilled hole" type of bony defect. These usually occur in the pelvis, distal femur, and spine. Highly comminuted fractures typically are caused by high-energy gunshots. The extent of bone comminution corresponds directly with the amount of the missile energy transferred and also suggests the degree of soft-tissue injury. Occasionally, fractures can be caused secondarily by the victim's fall after the shot. The severity of bone injury caused by gunshot is determined by the ability to maintain physiologic alignment and stability. Spine fractures due to gunshot rarely result in instability.

Risk of Infection Secondary to Gunshot Injury

Missiles projected from firearms are not sterile.[32] Some bacteria accumulated before the discharge of the missile can remain at the point of tissue impact,[33] although wound contamination occurs primarily from the skin flora, clothing, or any other material that may be encountered in the missile path. Although the risk of infection following typical civilian gunshot is rather low, injuries caused by bullets that traverse grossly contaminated areas such as large bowel carry exceptionally high infection risks. Also, high-energy gunshot injuries, in contrast to low-energy counterparts, are extremely prone to infection because of the greater soft-tissue damage and the presence of devitalized tissue debris. The extent of local contamination and presence of devitalized debris are critical in determining the optimal treatment approach.

GUNSHOT INJURY TO THE THORACOLUMBAR SPINE NEURAL ELEMENTS

Following a gunshot, the neural elements of the spine may be injured directly by perforating or penetrating missiles, indirectly by displaced bone fragments, or remotely by shock waves generated by high-energy missiles. Other injuring mechanisms can include a gunshot-induced disruption of the blood supply to the spinal cord and its structures, or as a consequence of loss of spinal stability and/or alignment. The direct violation of the spinal cord by perforating missiles with tearing of the dura and transection of the cord (total or subtotal) occurs over several spinal segments. In cases of penetrating missiles, the direct violation of spinal cord structures is further complicated by the bullet's presence in the spinal canal, which acts as a space-occupying mass.[34] Hematoma and fibrous scarring, precipitated by this mass, may cause supplemental injury.[35] A retained bullet in the canal can result in late complications related to the bullet migration,[36-40] lead poisoning,[41,42] neurotoxicity (copper-jacketed or brass-jacketed bullets),[31] and inflammatory foreign body reaction.[43]

Indirect mechanisms damage the cord by the displacing bone fragments created by the missile, or as a result of spinal instability. These mechanisms usually cause neurologic deficit by cord compression, and more closely resemble the damage usually observed in blunt trauma cord injury. Unlike blunt insults, high-energy missiles can remotely cause extensive neurologic damage at the level of the impact and/or extend over a distance above and below even without making contact with the spinal cord. In an animal model, high-energy gunshot injury to the spinous process of T12 or L1 produced complete neurologic deficits in all cases[44] by pressure shock waves propagated remotely from the missile track. The acoustic properties of the vertebrae can concentrate and propagate pressure waves into localized regions. Neural tissue appears to be extremely sensitive to the pressure waves created by gunshot injury.

The sensitivity of neural elements to direct or indirect insults places the cord and its related structures at extreme risk with both high-energy and low-energy injuries. With direct impact, the cord injury is usually well circumscribed and most severe at the site of the insult. Gross pathology may range from small superficial defects, to localized punctures, to incomplete or total cord transection with varying degrees of cerebral spinal fluid extravasation. When the missile traverses the thoracic spinal canal, a complete neurologic deficit almost always occurs.[11] Gunshot injuries in the lumbar spine may produce only partial neurologic deficits. Due to indirect mechanisms, remote lesions consisting of edema, necrosis, and/or hemorrhage may still occur throughout the cord. The neurologic injury level tends to be at least one segment higher than the vertebral injury level, while the sensory injury level is usually equal to or below the motor level of injury.[11,12] The spinal cord is also especially sensitive to ischemic changes, and gunshot injuries that disrupt the blood vessels supplying the cord usually result in pronounced neurologic deficit.

PATTERNS OF NEUROLOGIC DEFICIT

Thoracolumbar spine injuries due to gunshot may involve a variety of neural elements to include the spinal cord, nerve roots, the conus medullaris, and the cauda equina. The severity of neurologic deficits secondary to gunshot injuries differs from blunt spinal trauma[10] (Table 1). Among thoracolumbar spine gunshot injuries with neurologic deficits, complete neurologic deficits are more common than incomplete.[5,11,13,45-47] One report noted that approximately 75% of those with a spinal cord gunshot injury present with a complete neurologic deficit (Frankel grade A) on their initial neurologic examination. Waters and Adkins[5] reported that this complete neurologic deficit did not change at 1-year follow-up examination in two thirds of their patients. Among the one third of patients who did improve by one or two neurologic levels, the injury sustained primarily involved the cauda equina.

Yashon and associates[8] categorized spine gunshot injury patients into four groups according to their neurologic status: (1) immediate and complete clinical loss of spinal cord function; (2) incomplete nonprogressive spinal cord deficit; (3) incomplete, but progressive spinal cord deficit; and (4) injuries of the conus medullaris or cauda equina with neurologic deficit of varying severity. Among these groups, the authors noted that groups 1 and 4 were the most common. The authors also observed that the initial neurologic level may ascend one or two levels several days following injury; however, a complete neurologic deficit did not improve regardless of the treatment regimen used.[8] These findings were corroborated by Isiklar and

TABLE 1

Characteristics of Spinal Cord Injury Following Gunshot Injury Versus Nonviolent Trauma		
	Injury from Gunshot (% of patients)	Injury from Blunt Trauma (% of patients)
Paraplegia	78.0	48.8
Level of injury		
T1-T6	22.0	16.5
T7-T12	36.5	18.1
L1-L5	19.5	14.2
Frankel grade		
A	56.1	36.7
B	17.1	17.9
C	17.1	17.3
D	9.7	25.8
E	0.0	2.3

(Adapted with permission from McKinley WO, Johns JS, Musgrove JJ: Clinical presentations, medical complications, and functional outcomes of individuals with gunshot wound-induced spinal cord injury. *Am J Phys Med Rehabil* 1999;78:102-107.)

Lindsey[15] in their more recent review of patients who sustained a gunshot injury to the spine; they reported that patients with complete neurologic deficit on presentation demonstrated no long-term improvement.

THE INITIAL PATIENT ASSESSMENT

Patient History and Physical Examination

Patient evaluation following gunshot injury to the thoracolumbar spine should begin with a thorough history and clinical evaluation. Pertinent aspects of the history include the type of weapon, type of bullet, and its trajectory. This information may be the best early indication of the injury severity to the spine and its surrounding structures. Except for excessive bleeding, the wound should not be explored outside of the operating room due to the risk of increased morbidity.[48] The initial physical examination should determine the location of all entrance and exit wounds, and these wounds should be assessed to establish the extent of local soft-tissue injury and the path of the bullet. The tho-

FIGURE 1

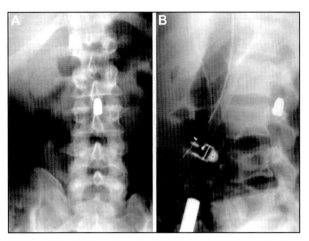

AP (**A**) and lateral (**B**) radiographs depicting gunshot injury to the lumbar spine with bullet retention. (Reproduced with permission from Isiklar ZU, Lindsey RW: Low-velocity civilian gunshot wounds of the spine. *Orthopedics* 1997;20:967-972.)

FIGURE 2

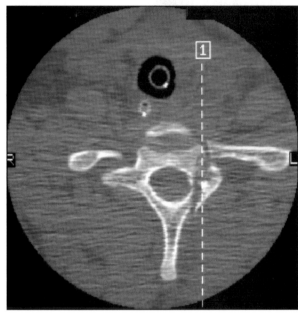

CT can be very useful for establishing bullet trajectory.

racolumbar spine is in close proximity to both the chest and the abdomen, and these cavities warrant careful evaluation.

The initial evaluation should include a comprehensive neurologic assessment. The neurologic examination should be performed and documented according to the Frankel Scale[49] or the American Spinal Injury Association (ASIA) Impairment Score.[50] The clinician should specifically establish if neurologic deficit is present or not, and if present, whether the deficit is complete versus incomplete. This can be reliably accomplished only after spinal shock has resolved as confirmed by the return of the bulbocavernosus reflex. Neurologic deficit may not occur at the level of bony injury.[51] In the thoracolumbar spine, the neural transition from cord to conus, and ultimately to cauda equina can challenge the precise documentation of neurologic injury that is necessary to determine the subsequent treatment and prognosis.

Imaging

Radiographic imaging is crucial to the evaluation process, and the minimum study consists of lateral spine views. These images can assist in localizing the spinal segments involved and determining the associated structures at risk (Figure 1). Patients with visualized spinal column injury or neurologic deficit without radiograph should also be evaluated with CT to more precisely determine the extent and location of injury as well as the presence of retained bullet or bone fragments.[52] CT is also helpful in more accurately determining the bullet track (Figure 2) and/or bullet location (Figure 3). Even in the presence of neurologic deficit, MRI of the thoracolumbar spine is usually contraindicated. Ferromagnetism of the missile can produce artifacts and image obscurity as well as induce deflection of the bullet and possibly cause additional injury.[53] Although it has been suggested that an MRI better delineates relationship between retained bullet in the cord than CT,[54] the information provided by MRI rarely influences outcome. In selected cases of cord injury without retained missile fragments, MRI may complement CT by better characterizing the extent of spinal cord injury.[55]

Although spinal stability is often thought to be maintained following gunshot injury to the spine, the recent clinical experience has suggested otherwise.[15] In the conscious, cooperative, and medically stable patient suspected of late thoracolumbar instability, voluntary lateral thoracolumbar flexion and extension are reasonable. However, dynamic imaging is rarely indicated in the acute setting.

INITIAL TREATMENT

The treatment of patients with gunshot injury to the thoracolumbar spine should adhere to the standard algo-

FIGURE 3

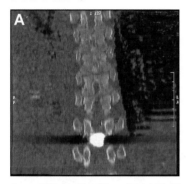
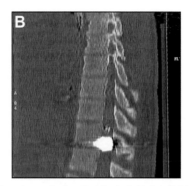
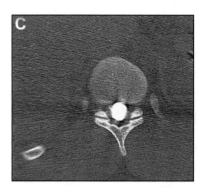

Coronal (**A**), sagittal (**B**), and axial (**C**) CT projections demonstrating that the bullet is located in the spinal canal. (Reproduced with permission from Lindsey RW, Gugala Z: Spinal cord injury as a result of ballistic trauma, in Chapman JR (ed): *Spine: State of the Art Reviews Spinal Cord Injuries.* Philadelphia, PA, Hanley & Belfus, 1999, vol 13, pp 529-547.)

rithm depicted in Figure 4. The first priority in the treatment of gunshot injuries to the thoracolumbar spine is the general medical condition of the patient.[15,26,56] If the patient is medically unstable, this suggests the presence of a visceral or vascular injury, which constitutes an emergency. Visceral injuries associated with thoracolumbar spine gunshot injuries can affect multiple structures and systems to include the pulmonary, cardiac, abdominal viscera, urinary, or major vessels. During initial treatment, all standard precautions should be used to protect the spine from additional injury (ie, backboard, sandbags, and maintaining the patient in a supine position). At this juncture, aside from an assessment of the patient's neurologic status, all efforts should be focused on stabilizing the patient's potentially life-threatening injuries.

Pharmacologic Management

Antibiotics

Patients with gunshot injuries to the thoracolumbar spine should receive high-dose parenteral broad-spectrum antibiotics and tetanus prophylaxis at presentation. Broad-spectrum antibiotic therapy to include coverage for gram-negative and anaerobic organisms is especially warranted for high-energy wounds or gunshot injuries in which the bowel is perforated.

Steroids

The primary gunshot injury (mechanical) to the spinal cord can be potentiated by the secondary mechanisms (biochemical) that form the premise for the administration of steroids. In blunt spinal cord injury, it has been shown that all of the damage to the spinal cord does not occur with the initial trauma, but continues with persistent compression.[57] However, the administration of steroids for gunshot spinal cord injury is highly controversial as presently there are no prospective randomized studies to justify their clinical use. Recent retrospective studies have failed to demonstrate neurologic recovery with steroid administration for ballistic spinal cord injury, and moreover, these studies suggest that steroids in this setting can be extremely hazardous.[58-61] These patients have been shown to be at significantly greater risk for infection or gastrointestinal complications[61] (Table 2).

Surgical Management

Surgery for Neurologic Deficit

When the patient is medically stable, the subsequent treatment is determined by the patient's neurologic status. In the presence of a complete neurologic deficit, surgery is not indicated, as the literature to date suggests that surgical decompression will not affect the ultimate neurologic outcome. Thoracolumbar spine decompression for gunshot-related neurologic deficit has not only proven to be ineffective, but may be detrimental. Stauffer and associates[62] studied 185 patients with complete neurologic deficits following spine gunshot injuries who were treated with surgical decompression. Decompression not only failed to improve the neurologic status of these patients, but also resulted in a multitude of other complications to include instability, infection, and spinal fluid fistula.[62]

Complete neurologic lesions involving the cauda equina may experience some degree of spontaneous resolution, especially when the injury is due to a low-energy

FIGURE 4

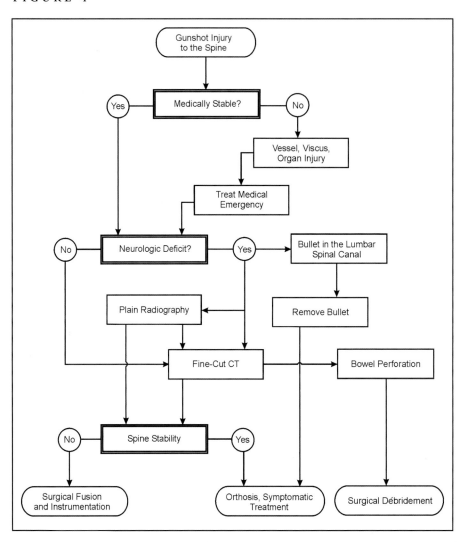

The authors' preferred management algorithm for patients with gunshot injury to the thoracolumbar spine.

gunshot wound. Stauffer and associates[62] reported a 94% improvement in patients with cauda equina neurologic deficits treated nonsurgically. Benzel and associates[45] reported improved recovery of nerve root function in all patients with cauda equina gunshot injuries with or without surgery. Isiklar and Lindsey[63] retrospectively studied 37 patients with low-energy gunshot injuries to the spine and further corroborated that neurologic recovery of one or two Frankel grades could be realized in patients with cauda equina injuries.

The presence of a missile fragment in proximity to neural elements may constitute a relative indication for decompression and bullet explantation. A collaborated study was performed by the National Spinal Cord Injury Model Systems, and consisted of serial neurologic examinations of 66 patients with bullet fragments impinging on neural elements. This prospective series suggested that patients with gunshot-related neurologic deficits can experience significant neurologic recovery, if the bullet was removed from the T12-L4 spinal segments.[5] Therefore, the neurologic anatomy of the thoracolumbar region may exhibit a more favorable response to surgical decompression for those patients sustaining low-energy gunshot injuries.[5,64] The optimal timing for decompression is unclear, but should be at least delayed until spinal shock has resolved. An absolute indication for immediate decompression would be a patient's

TABLE 2

Complications of Steroid Administration in Patients With Gunshot Injury to the Spine					
		Spinal Infection %	Extraspinal Infection %	Gastrointestinal Complications %	Pancreatitis %
No steroids	(n = 193)	2.6	16.1	2.6	5.2
Methylprednisolone	(n = 31)	3.2	25.8	0	16.1
Decamethasone	(n = 30)	10	20	13.3	0
Combined steroids	(n = 61)	6.6	23	6.6	-8.2

(Adapted with permission from Heary RF, Vaccaro AR, Mesa JJ, Balderston RA, Cotler JM: Steroids and gunshot injury to the spine. *Neurosurgery* 1997;41:576-583.)

sudden neurologic deterioration in the presence of clear neural element compromise from the gunshot injury.

If the gunshot injury to the thoracolumbar spine does not present with neurologic deficit, the indication for surgical interventions would be predicated on the risk for complications associated with retention of the bullet or the presence of spinal instability.

Surgery for Retained Missile Fragments
Bullet removal is rarely necessary following thoracolumbar spine gunshot injuries. Missile fragments that are lodged within the vertebral body, in the posterior elements, or have traversed through the spine and into the surrounding soft tissue are usually not problematic. The relative indications for missile removal would include a missile (or secondary bone fragments) lodged within the spinal canal that may cause late neurologic deficit, the missile that has perforated the alimentary canal before entering the spine, or the bullet at risk for causing toxicity. Missile fragments (both bullet and bone) that significantly compromise the spinal canal can threaten the patient's neurologic function, especially when located at the hypermobile thoracolumbar junction.[36,38,65] Early semielective excision of these fragments has been shown to improve motor recovery with conus medullaris and/or cauda equina injuries.[5,47,66] When missile fragments are not at risk for causing neural compromise, periodic radiographic evaluation is recommended. Retained bullet fragments may migrate and thereby cause late neurologic deficits.[37,38,67,68]

Surgery for Débridement
The incidence of infection after the spine gunshot injury is low and usually occurs in patients who have experi-

enced perforation of the alimentary tract before the missile enters the spine. The indications for early surgical intervention in the thoracolumbar spine are especially clear when the bullet has perforated large bowel or hollow viscera. Romanick and associates[29] reported that seven out of eight patients with spinal gunshot injuries associated with colon perforation developed infections despite antibiotic prophylaxis and concluded that early aggressive surgical débridement was warranted.

However, the indications for surgical débridement in these patients are also controversial. Roffi and associates[46] studied 35 spine gunshot injury patients with associated alimentary canal perforations among whom 18 were not surgically débrided. Despite the presence of colon perforations in 9 of the 18 nonsurgical patients, none of these patients developed an infection. The authors attributed their results to the sustained use of broad-spectrum intravenous antibiotics for up to 14 days and recommended administration of antibiotics for gram-negative and anaerobic organisms be maintained for several weeks. In another clinical series,[15] only one thoracolumbar spine gunshot injury became infected; this patient had sustained a colon perforation that was only treated with antibiotic regimen as recommended by Roffi and associates.[46] Currently, the authors recommend that strong consideration be given to the earlier surgical débridement of thoracolumbar spine gunshot injuries complicated by large bowel perforation.

Spinal Instability Following Gunshot Injury
Spinal instability secondary to low-energy gunshot injuries occurs infrequently, and the majority of thoracolumbar gunshot injuries can be treated with only an orthosis.

Historically, most of the reported cases of instability secondary to spine gunshot injuries have been iatrogenic as a result of an ill-advised surgical decompression.[62] However, Denis[69] reported a case of lumbar spine instability following gunshot injury, and Isiklar and Lindsey[15] reported gunshot-related lumbar instability despite appropriate immobilization. These authors concluded that although spinal stability following gunshot injuries is common, it is not necessarily guaranteed. This is especially the case in the more hypermobile thoracolumbar region of the spine. Therefore, the patients with thoracolumbar gunshot injuries should initially be placed in an appropriate orthotic support or brace, and be closely monitored until sufficient spinal stability has been established.

Significant comminution of the entire vertebral body poses a special concern as it increases the risk for spinal collapse and/or pronounced angular deformity. If surgical intervention to establish stability is warranted, techniques that limit the number of motion segments stabilized are preferred as the extent of instability is usually limited to the motion segment that has been injured. Furthermore, extensive decompression of the traumatized segments should be avoided (unless otherwise indicated) as this may only further destabilize the spine. Usually, posterior instrumentation alone will suffice. However, in the case of extensive comminution of both anterior and middle columns, an anterior procedure may be more appropriate. Techniques that consist of "front and back" stabilization are rarely indicated.

Lead Toxicity

The risk for lead toxicity would justify early surgical débridement, however, this complication is rarely encountered. Lead dissolution typically occurs when the bullet is in contact with synovial fluid, a pseudocyst, or a disk space.[42,67,70] The patient will usually require prolonged exposure to the bullet before experiencing lead poisoning symptoms such as abdominal pain, anemia, headaches, memory loss, and muscle weakness. When this phenomenon occurs, medical treatment consisting of chelation therapy with EDTA (ethylenediaminetetraacetate), D-penicillamine, or dimercaptol may prove effective even before the eventual bullet removal.[63]

Conclusions

Gunshot injuries to the spine constitute the second most common cause of spinal cord injury. Therefore, it is imperative for the clinician to be familiar with the distinctions of the penetrating versus blunt spine injuries. The clinician should appreciate the ballistic principles of missile wounding, and be able to clinically determine gunshot injury severity. At presentation, patients with gunshot injuries to the spine receive parenteral broad-spectrum antibiotics and tetanus prophylaxis. As opposed to blunt spine trauma patients, in penetrating spine trauma with neurologic deficit steroids are not indicated. Spinal decompression has not proven to be effective for gunshot injuries, and should be reserved for cases in which progressive neurologic deficit or cauda equina injuries exist. Spinal débridement in combination with broad-spectrum antibiotics should be considered in patients with concomitant large bowel perforation. Spinal gunshot injury rarely results in spinal instability; however, the patient warrants careful monitoring until stability has been clearly established.

References

1. Schwab CW: Members of the Violence Prevention Task Force of the Eastern Association for the Surgery of Trauma: Violence in America. A public health crisis: The role of firearms. *J Trauma* 1995;38:163-168.
2. Wintemute GJ: The relationship between firearm design and firearm violence: Handguns in the 1990s. *JAMA* 1996;275:1749-1753.
3. Carrillo EH, Gonzalez JK, Carrillo LE, et al: Spinal cord injuries in adolescents after gunshot wounds: An increasing phenomenon in urban North America. *Injury* 1998;29:503-507.
4. Schwab CW, Richmond T, Dunfey M: Firearm injury in America. *LDI Issue Brief* 2002;8:1-6.
5. Waters RL, Adkins RH: The effects of removal of bullet fragments retained in the spinal canal: A collaborative study by the National Spinal Cord Injury Model Systems. *Spine* 1991;16:934-939.
6. Waters RL, Sie IH: Spinal cord injuries from gunshot wounds to the spine. *Clin Orthop* 2003;408:120-125.
7. Yoshida GM, Garland D, Waters RL: Gunshot wounds to the spine. *Orthop Clin North Am* 1995;26:109-116.
8. Yashon D, Jane JA, White RJ: Prognosis and management of spinal cord and cauda equina bullet injuries in sixty-five civilians. *J Neurosurg* 1970;32:163-170.
9. Burney RE, Maio RF, Maynard F, Karunas R: Incidence, characteristics, and outcome of spinal cord injury at trauma centers in North America. *Arch Surg* 1993;128:596-599.
10. McKinley WO, Johns JS, Musgrove JJ: Clinical presentations, medical complications, and functional outcomes of

individuals with gunshot wound-induced spinal cord injury. *Am J Phys Med Rehabil* 1999;78:102-107.

11. Waters RL, Adkins RH, Yakura J, Sie I: Profiles of spinal cord injury and recovery after gunshot injury. *Clin Orthop* 1991;267:14-21.

12. Waters RL, Sie IH, Adkins RH: Rehabilitation of a patient with a spinal cord injury. *Orthop Clin North Am* 1995;26:117-122.

13. Kane T, Capen D, Waters R, Zigler JE, Adkins R: Spinal cord injury from civilian gunshot wounds: The Rancho experience 1980-88. *J Spinal Disord* 1991;4:306-311.

14. Eismont FJ: Gunshot wounds to the spine, in Levine AM, Eismont FJ, Garfin SR, Zigler JE (eds): *Spine Trauma*. Philadelphia, PA, WB Saunders, 1998, pp 525-543.

15. Isiklar ZU, Lindsey RW: Low-velocity civilian gunshot wounds of the spine. *Orthopedics* 1997;20:967-972.

16. Lindsey D: The idolatry, lies, damn lies, and ballistics. *J Trauma* 1980;20:1068-1069.

17. Fackler ML: Wound ballistics: A review of current misconceptions. *JAMA* 1988;259:2730-2736.

18. Fackler ML: Civilian gunshot wounds and ballistics: Dispelling the myths. *Emerg Med Clin North Am* 1998;16:17-28.

19. Adams BD: Wound ballistics: A review. *Mil Med* 1982;147:831-835.

20. Belkin M: Wound ballistics. *Prog Surg* 1979;16:7-24.

21. Shepard GH: High-energy, low-velocity close range shotgun wounds. *J Trauma* 1980;20:1065-1067.

22. Sherman RT, Parrish RA: Management of shotgun injuries: A review of 152 cases. *J Trauma* 1963;3:76-85.

23. Ordog GJ, Wasserberger J, Balasubramaniam S: Shotgun wound ballistics. *J Trauma* 1988;28:624-631.

24. Gugala Z, Lindsey RW: Classification of gunshot injuries in civilians. *Clin Orthop* 2003;408:65-81.

25. Shuman M, Wright RK: Evaluation of clinician accuracy in describing the gunshot wound injuries. *J Forensic Sci* 1999;44:339-342.

26. Lindsey RW, Gugala Z: Spinal cord injury as a result of ballistic trauma, in Chapman JR (ed): *Spine: State of the Art Reviews Spinal Cord Injuries*. Philadelphia, PA, Hanley & Belfus, 1999, vol 13, pp 529-547.

27. Primm DD: Lead arthropathy: Progressive destruction of the joint by a retained bullet. *J Bone Joint Surg Am* 1984;66:292-294.

28. Rhee JM, Martin R: The management of retained bullets in the limbs. *Injury* 1997;28(suppl 3):23-28.

29. Romanick PC, Smith TK, Kopaniky DR, Oldfield D: Infection about the spine associated with low-velocity-missile injury to the abdomen. *J Bone Joint Surg Am* 1985;67:1195-1201.

30. Sherman IJ: Brass foreign body in the brain stem. *J Neurosurg* 1960;17:483-485.

31. Messer HD, Cerza PF: Copper-jacketed bullets in the central nervous system. *Neuroradiology* 1976;12:121-129.

32. Thoresby FP, Darlow HM: The mechanisms of primary infection of bullet wounds. *Br J Surg* 1967;54:359-361.

33. Wolf AW, Benson DR, Shoji H, Hoeprich P, Gilmore A: Autosterilization in low-velocity bullets. *J Trauma* 1978;18:63.

34. Wigle RL: Treatment of asymptomatic gunshot injury to the spine. *Am Surg* 1989;55:591-595.

35. Weinshel S, Maiman D: Spinal subdural hematoma presenting as an epidural hematoma following gunshot: Report of a case. *J Spinal Disord* 1988;1:317-319.

36. Arasil E, Tascioglu AO: Spontaneous migration of an intracranial bullet to the cervical spinal canal causing Lhermitte's sign: A case report. *J Neurosurg* 1982;56:158-159.

37. Karim NO, Nabors MW, Golocovsky M, Cooney FD: Spontaneous migration of a bullet in the spinal subarachnoid space causing delayed radicular symptoms. *Neurosurgery* 1986;18:97-100.

38. Avci S, Acikgoz B, Gundogdu S: Delayed neurological symptoms from the spontaneous migration of a bullet in the lumbosacral spinal canal: Case report. *Paraplegia* 1995;33:541-542.

39. Oktem IS, Selcuklu A, Kurtsoy A, Kavuncu IA, Pasaoglu A: Migration of bullet in the spinal canal: A case report. *Surg Neurol* 1995;44:548-550.

40. Rajan DK, Alcantara AL, Michael DB: Where's the bullet? A migration in two acts. *J Trauma* 1997;43:716-718.

41. Dillman RO, Crumb CK, Lidsky MJ: Lead poisoning from a gunshot wound: Report of a case and review of the literature. *Am J Med* 1979;66:509-514.

42. Grogan DP, Bucholz RW: Acute lead intoxication from a bullet in an intervertebral disc space: A case report. *J Bone Joint Surg Am* 1981;63:1180-1182.

43. Daniel EF, Smith GW: Foreign body granuloma of intervertebral disc and spinal canal. *J Neurosurg* 1960;17:480-482.

44. De-Wen W, Zhun-Shan W, Xao-Gang Y, et al: Histologic and utrastructural changes of the spinal cord after high-velocity missile injury to the back. *J Trauma* 1996;40:90-93.

45. Benzel EC, Hadden TA, Coleman JE: Civilian gunshot wounds to the spinal cord and cauda equina. *Neurosurgery* 1987;20:281-285.

46. Roffi RP, Waters RL, Adkins RH: Gunshot wounds to the spine associated with a perforated viscus. *Spine* 1989;14:808-811.

47. Kihtir T, Ivatury RR, Simon R, Stahl WM: Management of transperitoneal gunshot wounds of the spine. *J Trauma* 1991;31:1579-1583.

48. Golueke P, Scalfari S, Philips T, Goldstein A, Scalea T, Duncan A: Vertebral artery injury diagnosis and management. *J Trauma* 1987;27:856-865.

49. Frankel HL, Hancock DO, Hyslop G, et al: The value of postural reduction in the initial management of closed injuries of the spine with paraplegia and tetraplegia. *Paraplegia* 1969;7:179-192.

50. American Spinal Cord Injury Association: *International Standards for Neurological Classification of Spinal Cord Injuries.* New York, NY, Raven Press, 2002.

51. DeMuth WE Jr.: Bullet velocity and design and determinants of wounding capability: An experimental study. *J Trauma* 1969;6:222-232.

52. Plumley TF, Kilcoyne RF, Mack LA: Computed tomography in evaluation of gunshot wounds to the spine. *J Comput Assist Tomogr* 1983;7:310-312.

53. Teitelbaum GP: Metallic ballistic fragments: MR imaging safety and artifacts. *Radiology* 1990;177:883.

54. Ebraheim NA, Savolaine ER, Jackson WT, Andreshak TG, Rayport M: Magnetic resonance imaging in the evaluation of a gunshot wound to the cervical spine. *J Orthop Trauma* 1989;3:19-22.

55. Bashir EF, Cybulski GR, Chaudhri K, Choudhury AR: Magnetic resonance imaging and computed tomography in the evaluation of penetrating gunshot injury of the spine: Case report. *Spine* 1993;18:772-773.

56. Simpson R, Venger B, Narayan R: Treatment of acute penetrating injuries of the spine: A retrospective analysis. *J Trauma* 1989;29:42-46.

57. Delamarter RB, Sherman J, Carr JB: Pathophysiology of spinal cord injury: Recovery after immediate and delayed compression. *J Bone Joint Surg Am* 1995;77:1042-1049.

58. Prendergast MR, Saxe JM, Ledgerwood AM, Lucas CE, Lucas WF: Massive steroids do not reduce the zone of injury after penetrating spinal cord injury. *J Trauma* 1994;37:576-580.

59. Heary RF, Vaccaro AR, Mesa JJ, Balderston RA: Thoracolumbar infections in penetrating injuries to the spine. *Orthop Clin North Am* 1996;27:69-81.

60. Levy ML, Gans W, Wijesinghe HS, SooHoo WE, Adkins RH, Stillerman CB: Use of methylprednisolone as an adjunct in the management of patients with penetrating spinal cord injury: Outcome analysis. *Neurosurgery* 1996;39:1141-1148.

61. Heary RF, Vaccaro AR, Mesa JJ, et al: Steroids and gunshot wounds to the spine. *Neurosurgery* 1997;41:576-583.

62. Stauffer ES, Wood RW, Kelly EG: Gunshot wounds of the spine: The effects of laminectomy. *J Bone Joint Surg Am* 1979;61:389-392.

63. Isiklar ZU, Lindsey RW: Gunshot wounds to the spine. *Injury* 1998;29(suppl 1):SA7-SA12.

64. Cybulski GR, Sone JL, Kant R: Outcome of laminectomy for civilian gunshot injuries of the terminal spinal cord and cauda equina: Review of 88 cases. *Neurosurgery* 1989;24:392-397.

65. Conway JE, Crofford TW, Terry AF, Protzman RR: Cauda equina syndrome occurring nine years after gunshot injury to the spine. *J Bone Joint Surg Am* 1993;75:760-763.

66. Robertson DP, Simpson RK: Penetrating injuries restricted to the cauda equina: A retrospective review. *Neurosurgery* 1992;31:265-270.

67. Leonard MH: The solution of lead by synovial fluid. *Clin Orthop* 1969;64:255-261.

68. Tanguy A, Chabannes J, Deubelle A, Vanneuville G, Dalens B: Intraspinal migration of a bullet with subsequent meningitis. *J Bone Joint Surg Am* 1982;64:1244-1245.

69. Denis F: The three-column spine and its significance in the classification of acute thoracolumbar spine injuries. *Spine* 1983;8:817-831.

70. Linden MA, Manton WI, Stewart RM, Thal ER, Feit H: Lead poisoning from retained bullets: Pathogenesis, diagnosis, and management. *Ann Surg* 1982;195:305-313.

CHAPTER 11

MANAGEMENT OF OSTEOPOROTIC COMPRESSION FRACTURES

MICHAEL HEGGENESS, MD, PhD

Vertebral fractures associated with osteoporosis are common, but reliable prevalence and incidence rates are extremely difficult to estimate. Precise diagnostic criteria are also difficult to establish. Minor degrees of end plate collapse are often difficult to see on plain radiographs. Projectional artifact and the low mineral density of the bones contribute to the difficulty.[1] Classic epidemiologic studies have reported wide variations in the presentation and progression of vertebral collapse in osteoporosis, from which some general conclusions can be formed.[1-9] In general, the earliest fractures occur in the upper thoracic spine, many of which are asymptomatic. Progressive collapse of multiple vertebrae in this area often leads to a significant upper thoracic kyphosis, often referred to as a "dowager's hump."

Patients with these fractures frequently present with acute back pain but no initial radiographic evidence of fracture, which adds to the diagnostic challenge. Images taken days or weeks later often document vertebral collapse, a phenomenon that illustrates an important point about osteoporotic compression fractures: the fractured vertebra in these patients frequently demonstrates insidious, progressive collapse over weeks or months to a degree not seen in younger patients.

CLASSIFICATION

In the context of axial load, vertebral fractures are classified initially on the basis of the integrity of the posterior cortex (the "middle column") of the vertebral body (Figure 1). Fractures that involve the end plate and anterior cortex, but spare the posterior cortex, are called compression fractures. Those that also involve the posterior cortex are referred to as burst fractures. All burst fractures have the potential to increase morbidity given the possibility of associated nerve compression. This injury is often associated with retropulsion of bony fragments into the canal, which can cause neurologic deficit. In addition, when the posterior cortex is injured, the potential for collapse, angulation, and progression of deformity is much greater.

Most osteoporotic vertebral fractures result from failure under axial compression.[10,11] These injuries are commonly referred to as compression fractures, even though they quite frequently involve the posterior cortex. Thus, many of these fractures are, technically, true burst fractures. Very few of these fractures are imaged by CT or MRI; therefore, the true incidence of middle column injuries is not known. Classic anatomic studies have shown, however, that middle column failure is very common.[12,13]

Most attempts to classify vertebral fractures have been based on criteria established with plain radiographs. The classification system of Eastell and associates[14] has proved to be useful. Vertebral fractures are often referred to by their gross morphology as "biconcave" or "codfish" fractures, "wedge" fractures, or "crush" fractures. Crush fractures involve a gross failure of both cortices. However, the

FIGURE 1

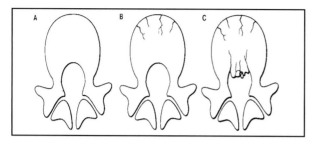

Axial views of the vertebral body. **A,** Normal vertebra. **B,** Compression fracture characterized by injury to the anterior cortex, resulting in loss of height. Note that the bony borders of the spinal canal are not affected. **C,** Burst fracture characterized by injury to the borders of the spinal canal. (Reproduced with permission from Heggeness MH, Mathis KB: An orthopaedic perspective of osteoporosis, in Marcus R, Feldman D, Kelsey J (eds): *Osteoporosis.* Philadephia, PA, Academic Press, 1996.)

percentage of biconcave or wedge fractures that also have some posterior cortical involvement is not known. Frequently, what appears to be an isolated end plate fracture may undergo progressive collapse, resulting in a wedge fracture and, ultimately, a crush fracture (or burst fracture) over days and weeks of observation. Rarely, this sequence of events can lead to devastating late neurologic dysfunction.[15-20]

MANAGEMENT

History and Physical Examination

Management of osteoporosis-related compression fractures includes investigation of other possible causes of pathologic fractures and, in most instances, nonsurgical treatment. The patient's history should include specific information regarding osteoporosis risk factors, such as a history of smoking or excessive alcohol intake, and a detailed surgical and medical history. The possibility of multiple myeloma must be kept in mind. A history of unexplained weight loss may be particularly suggestive of malignancy. Thus, radiographs should be carefully examined for fracture morphology. A history of previous fracture can be very useful in differentiating insufficiency fractures from those associated with malignancy.

Laboratory studies should include a complete blood cell count, urinalysis, serum calcium and phosphorus levels, and thyroid function tests. In an elderly Caucasian woman without evidence of other contributing history, a tentative diagnosis of osteoporosis may be considered if results

of these studies are within normal limits. Men or young women with osteoporosis may require additional workup and endocrinologic consultation. A careful neurologic examination, particularly of the lower extremities, is mandatory. A general physical examination should include a breast examination and palpation of the thyroid. The presence of objective neurologic dysfunction presents a strong indication for CT or MRI.

Patient Education and Pain Management

Patient education must be included as part of initial management. It is important for the patient to understand the diagnosis and its implications. The possibility of subsequent fracture also should be discussed, although it is important to stress that vertebral fractures heal successfully in almost all cases and that spontaneous resolution of pain may be expected in 2 to 10 weeks, regardless of treatment. Patients are advised to seek prompt medical attention should neurologic signs or symptoms develop.

Pain management is a critical concern to these patients. When pain is inadequately controlled, many patients become sedentary, often confining themselves to bed rest, which increases their risk for venous thrombosis and progression of their osteoporosis. The exact effect of prolonged bed rest on bone mineral density in patients with osteoporosis has not been studied. However, bed rest studies on younger patients indicate that bone loss of up to 1% a week can be expected.[21] On this basis, the authors strongly discouraged bed rest and suggested patient mobilization as a critical aspect of care. A short course of oral narcotic analgesics is often indicated to allow patients a reasonable level of activity.

Nonsurgical Treatment

The use of braces for treatment of an acute fracture is controversial. Many elderly patients, despite their pain, cannot tolerate a brace. Any attempt to brace fractures in the upper thoracic spine is particularly difficult and too rarely successful for pain management. Simple braces, such as canvas corsets, can be extremely useful for lumbar fractures and often afford a dramatic level of pain relief. Bracing thoracolumbar and midthoracic fractures is more difficult because a lumbosacral corset often does not provide adequate support to this region. Many patients with thoracolumbar fractures find significant relief with a custom-molded, soft-foam brace.

The use of braces for these problems remains an ongoing controversy because of the theoretical possibility that stress shielding of the spine may occur, exacerbating the osteoporosis. In my experience, patients with osteoporosis will use a brace only so long as it is useful for severe pain management; thus, the benefits of keeping the patient ambulatory may outweigh potential risks of stress shielding. Unfortunately, no firm data are available on which to form a firm conclusion. A few patients will experience such severe pain and physical limitation from fracture that hospitalization is required for supportive care and parenteral pain medication. Mobilization of these patients, even when hospitalized, is encouraged.

Use of parenteral calcitonin is gaining acceptance in the acute management of vertebral compression fractures. For unknown reasons, many patients who sustain vertebral compression fractures obtain dramatic analgesia from the use of calcitonin. While the basis of the phenomenon may lie in the documented central nervous system receptors for this hormone, its precise mode of action in analgesia remains unknown. Parenteral doses of calcitonin of approximately 100 IU/day are extremely effective in providing pain relief for some patients. However, hypersensitivity reactions have been described, and many patients experience transient gastrointestinal symptoms of nausea and vomiting during the initial days of therapy. Because of these unpleasant side effects, smaller doses are usually given initially (5 to 20 IU), and the dosage is slowly increased into the therapeutic range over 3 to 5 days. Symptomatic treatment of nausea is often helpful during this interval. A nasal spray form of calcitonin is also available for analgesic purposes. However, in my experience, the subcutaneous administration is much more effective.

Calcitonin treatment and external bracing usually can be discontinued within 4 to 10 weeks of the fracture event. Unfortunately, some patients experience relentless occurrence of multiple vertebral fractures through their sixth, seventh, and eighth decades of life. Dramatic kyphotic deformity and severe postural impairments often result. Chronic back pain with associated degenerative disease and kyphosis can be an extremely frustrating problem.

Progression of kyphosis usually stops when the lower ribs begin to impinge on the iliac wings. Unfortunately, localized pain typically develops as a result of irritation of soft tissues and costal nerves in this area. In rare cases, severe intractable pain may be managed by costal nerve blocks. Spinal osteotomy, rib resection, and multiple level spinal fusions are discouraged.

SPINE FRACTURE WITH NEUROLOGIC DEFICIT

The literature suggests that while the incidence of vertebral fractures in the aging population is high, neurologic dysfunction from these fractures occurs in only extremely rare cases. Reports of patients with neurologic dysfunction have appeared with much greater frequency in recent years, however, and it is likely that this phenomenon is more common than has been previously appreciated.[15-17,19,20]

All reports described the common characteristics of the clinical presentation of these injuries. In nearly every case, fractures occurred either spontaneously or after minor trauma. The initial presentation involved a report of back pain only. Patients subsequently experience progressive, insidious collapse of the fractured vertebra, followed by radicular pain and neurologic deficit weeks or months after the initial fracture event (Figure 2). I believe that radicular pain always precedes the development of motor deficit.

The development of neurologic symptoms is an acceptable indication to consider surgical intervention. Shakata and associates,[18] Kaneda and associates,[19] and others have advocated aggressive surgical decompression and stabilization of these injuries. These authors report that nonsurgical treatment, specifically physical therapy, can also provide excellent results in patients with relatively minor deficits. In patients with major neurologic deficits and dramatic motor dysfunction, however, surgical management, while difficult, is generally recommended. These patients are frequently elderly and often have comorbidities associated with smoking, alcohol use, or other complicating illnesses. Thus, surgical options for these patients must be individualized.

In general, surgical intervention consists of an anterior approach to the spine, corpectomy, and reconstruction. I favor anterior instrumentation, although simultaneous or staged posterior stabilization also may be appropriate, depending on surgeon preference and the individual clinical situation. Iliac crest autograft struts, as well as allograft and ceramic spacers, may have a role in the surgical treatment. Instrumentation of the anterior spine in severely osteopenic patients requires meticulous technique and the creation of a construct with load sharing between nonfractured posterior elements, the bone graft itself, and the instrumentation system.

I personally favor screw rod systems for instrumentation of these fractures, as the screw placement site is not constrained as much as with screw plate devices[22] (Figure

FIGURE 2

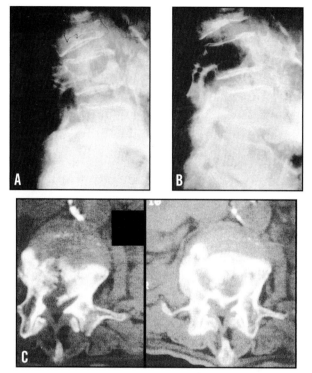

Radiographic evidence of progressive, insidious vertebral collapse seen in an 82-year-old patient who reported weakness and back and leg pain on presentation. **A,** Lateral view obtained 3 weeks after the onset of back pain. **B,** Follow-up lateral view of the same patient 3 weeks later. Note the continued loss of height shown in this L2 fracture. **C,** CT scans show bony fragments within the spinal canal. The patient was treated non-surgically with a brace and analgesics and made a complete recovery. (Reproduced with permission from Heggeness MH, Mathis KB: An orthopaedic perspective of osteoporosis, in Marcus R, Feldman D, Kelsey J (eds): *Osteoporosis*. Philadephia, PA, Academic Press, 1996.)

FIGURE 3

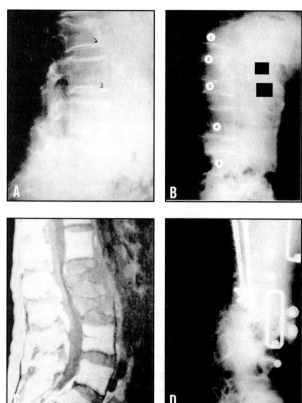

Radiographic evidence of insidious vertebral collapse of a fracture of L2 seen in an osteoporotic 78-year-old patient following a minor fall. **A,** Lateral view obtained immediately after the incident. **B,** Follow-up lateral view obtained 7 weeks later. Note the profound collapse of L2 and the fracture of the body of L3. At the time this radiograph was obtained, the patient reported severe leg pain and had profound motor deficits. **C,** MRI scan shows disruption of the borders of the vertebral canal, with bony fragments impinging the neural elements. Surgical treatment ensued, consisting of an anterior approach to the spine, débridement of the fracture with decompression of the neural elements, bone grafting, and anterior instrumentation. **D,** Postoperative lateral view shows Kostuik-Harrington rods in place.

3). Extended biomechanical studies have not addressed the question of the relative advantage of different screw designs. However, large cancellous threads would seem to offer some advantage in this situation. Bicortical technique is also advised because it adds substantially to the bio-mechanical stability of the screws.[23]

Biomechanical studies of posterior instrumentation techniques have suggested that hook constructs may offer some advantage over pedicle screw constructs in osteoporotic patients,[24] although specific techniques such as rigid cross-linking and hook screw constructs leave many options for the surgeon to individualize treatment (Figure 4).

My experience suggests that the clinical phenomenon of neurologic deficit from osteoporosis-related spine fracture is prob-ably a good deal more common than is generally appreciated. The insidious presentation of the neurologic deficits frequently leads to a missed or delayed diagnosis. Increased awareness of this injury may lead to more prompt and accurate diagnosis and, it is to be hoped, more appropriate treatment.

Late follow-up of patients treated nonsurgically whose neurologic deficit has resolved reveals progressive resorption and remodeling of the compressive bone fragments within the spinal canal, although the resorption occurs much more slowly than the clinically observed neurologic recovery.

FIGURE 4

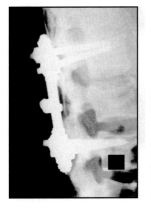

Lateral radiograph shows posterior instrumentation and stabilization of an L3 fracture. (Reproduced with permission from Heggeness MH, Mathis KB: An orthopaedic perspective of osteoporosis, in Marcus R, Feldman D, Kelsey J (eds): *Osteoporosis.* Philadelphia, PA, Academic Press, 1996.)

POLYMETHYLMETHACRYLATE BONE AUGMENTATION PROCEDURES

Osteoporosis-related compression fractures can be treated by injection of polymerizing methylmethacrylate bone cement. This technique has been in use for over 20 years. Recently, with the development of more sophisticated cement injection technology, methylmethacrylate injection for the treatment of acute and subacute vertebral fractures has gained enormous popularity. However, there are two commonly used techniques for methylmethacrylate injection: vertebroplasty and kyphoplasty.

Vertebroplasty involves the percutaneous introduction of a cannula or sleeve into the interior of the vertebral body (Figure 5). This procedure can be done under general or local anesthesia. Polymethylmethacrylate is then injected into the vertebral body and allowed to cure within the vertebral body. This is thought to provide mechanical stability to the fractured bone and appears to result in excellent and immediate pain relief.[25-30] Biomechanical studies confirming the proposed mechanical effects of the cement have not yet emerged. Another possible explanation for the clinically observed pain relief may be related to thermal or chemical ablation.[31,32] More research is needed on this subject.

Kyphoplasty is similar to vertebroplasty in that it involves injection of methylmethacrylate for fracture stabilization. However, with kyphoplasty, the methylmethacrylate injection is preceded by the inflation of two paired plastic balloons within these central areas of the vertebral body (Figure 6). This creates a cavity for the cement to fill and is thought

FIGURE 5

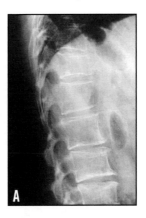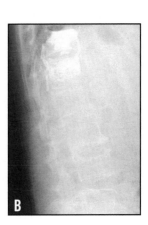

Radiographs of a two-level vertebroplasty performed on a 72-year-old patient with osteoporosis. **A,** Preoperative lateral view. **B,** Postoperative lateral view.

FIGURE 6

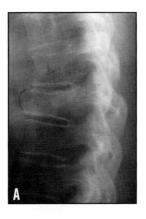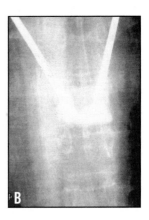

Radiographs of a kyphoplasty performed on a 68-year-old patient with a fracture of T7. Note that the patient was also steroid dependent. **A,** Preoperative lateral view. **B,** Intraoperative PA view.

to, in some cases, allow reduction (restoration of height) of the fractured end plates. Early reports on the clinical use of kyphoplasty indicate similar, very encouraging rates of pain relief, although there is some controversy about the efficiency of the end plate reduction portion of this procedure.

The two techniques are technically challenging. Accurate placement of the methylmethacrylate delivery system is essential. Injury of vessels, nerve roots, and other anatomically important structures is possible in the process of introducing the device into the vertebral body.

Further, methylmethacrylate injection can result in extravasation of methacrylate into adjacent structures such as the great vessels, nerve roots, and the spinal canal. Additionally, methylmethacrylate embolization and toxicities from methylmethacrylate monomer causing heart arrhythmias are reported. To use these techniques safely, excellent high-resolution fluoroscopy equipment is necessary. The community is unanimous in supporting the contention that experience and great caution are necessary to perform this technique safely.

SUMMARY AND CONCLUSIONS

Thoracolumbar fractures in patients with osteoporosis can present difficult clinical challenges. Fortunately, the overwhelming majority of such fractures respond to nonsurgical management. The prevention of future fractures is also important, including counseling the patient regarding appropriate medication as well as measures to take to prevent falls in the home.

REFERENCES

1. Cooper C, Atkinson EJ, O'Fallon WM, Melton LJ III: Incidence of clinically diagnosed vertebral fractures: A population-based study in Rochester, Minnesota, 1985-1989. *J Bone Miner Res* 1992;7:221-227.

2. Urist MR, Gurvey MS, Fareed DO: Long term observations on aged women with pathologic osteoporosis, in *Osteoporosis*. New York, NY, Grune & Stratton, 1970, pp 3-37.

3. Saville PD: Observations on 80 women with osteoporotic spine fractures, in *Osteoporosis*. New York, NY, Grune & Stratton, 1970, pp 38-46.

4. Kanis JA, Pitt FA: Epidemiology of osteoporosis. *Bone* 1992;13:S7-S15.

5. Iskrant AP, Smith RW: Osteoporosis in women 45 years and over related to subsequent fractures. *Public Health Rep* 1969;84:33-38.

6. Melton LJ III, Kan SH, Frye MA, Wagner HW, O'Fallon WMN, Riggs BL: Epidemiology of vertebral fractures during 30 years. *Am J Epidemiol* 1989;42:293-296.

7. Bengner U, Johnell O, Redlund-Johnell I: Changes in incidence and prevalence of vertebral fractures during 30 years. *Calcif Tissue Int* 1988;42:293-296.

8. Avioli LV: Significance of osteoporosis: A growing international health problem. *Calcif Tissue Int* 1991;49 (suppl):5-7.

9. Leidig G, Minne HW, Sauer P, et al: A study of complaints in their relation to vertebral destruction in patients with osteoporosis. *Bone Miner* 1990;8:217-229.

10. Denis F: The three column spine and its significance in the classification of acute thoracolumbar spinal injuries. *Spine* 1983;8:817-831.

11. Holdsworth FW: Fractures, dislocations and fracture dislocations of the spine. *J Bone Joint Surg Am* 1970;52:1534-1551.

12. Schmorl G, Junghans H: *The Human Spine in Health and Disease*. New York, NY, Grune & Stratton, 1971.

13. Jaffe HJ: *Metabolic Degenerative and Inflammatory Diseases of Bone and Joints*. Philadelphia, PA, Lea & Febiger, 1972.

14. Eastell R, Cedel SL, Wahner HW, Riggs BL, Melton LJ III: Classification of vertebral fractures. *J Bone Miner Res* 1991;6:207-215.

15. Arciero RA, Leung KYK, Pierce JH: Spontaneous unstable burst fracture of the thoracolumbar spine in osteoporosis: A report of two cases. *Spine* 1989;14:114-117.

16. Salomon C, Chopin D, Benoist M: Spinal cord compression: An exceptional complication of spinal osteoporosis. *Spine* 1988;13:222-224.

17. Tan SB, Kozak JA, Mawad ME: The limitations of magnetic resonance imaging in the diagnostic of pathologic vertebral fractures. *Spine* 1991;16:919-923.

18. Shakata J, Yamamuro T, Iida H, Shimizu K, Yoshikawa J: Surgical treatment of paraplegia resulting from vertebral fractures in senile osteoporosis. *Spine* 1990;15:485-489.

19. Kaneda K, Asano S, Hashimoto T, Satoh S, Fujiya M: The treatment of osteoporotic-posttraumatic vertebral collapse using the Kaneda device and a bioactive ceramic vertebral prosthesis. *Spine* 1992;17(suppl):S295-S303.

20. Heggeness MH: Spine fracture with neurological deficit in osteoporosis. *Osteoporos Int* 1993;3:215-221.

21. LeBlanc AD, Schneider VS, Evans HJ, Engelbretson DA, Krebs JM: Bone mineral loss and recovery after 17 weeks of reduction. *J Bone Miner Res* 1990;5:843-850.

22. Kostuik JP: Anterior fixation for burst fractures of the thoracic and lumbar spine with or without neurological involvement. *Spine* 1988;13:286-293.

23. Breeze SW, Doherty BJ, Nobel PS, LeBlanc A, Heggeness MH: A biomechanical study of anterior thoracolumbar screw fixation. *Spine* 1998;23:1829-1831.

24. Coe JD, Warden KE, Herzig MA, McAfee PC: Influence of bone mineral density on the fixation of thoracolumbar implants. *Spine* 1988;15:902-907.

25. Martin JB, Jean B, Sugiu K, et al: Vertebroplasty: Clinical experience and follow-up results. *Bone* 1999;25(suppl 2):11S-15S.

26. Cortet B, Cotten A, Boutry N, et al: Percutanious vertebroplasty in the treatment of osteoporotic vertebral compression fractures: An open prospective study. *J Rheumatol* 1999;26:2222-2228.

27. Barr J, Barr M, Lemley T, McCann R: Percutaneous vertebroplasty for pain relief and spinal stabilization. *Spine* 2000;25:923-928.

28. Watts NB, Harris ST, Genant HK: Treatment of painful osteoporotic vertebral fractures with percutaneous vertebroplasty or kyphoplasty. *Osteoporos Int* 2001;12:429-437.

29. Lieberman IH, Dudeney S, Reinhardt MK, Bell G: Initial outcome of efficacy of "kyphoplasty" in the treatment of painful osteoporotic vertebral compression fractures. *Spine* 2001;26:1631-1638.

30. Garfin SR, Yan HA, Reiley MA: New technologies in spine: Kyphoplasty and vertebroplasty for the treatment of painful osteoporotic compression fractures. *Spine* 2001;26:1511-1515.

31. Antonacci MD, Mody DR, Rutz K, Weilbaecher D, Heggeness MH: A histologic study of fractured human vertebral bodies. *J Spinal Disord* 2002;15:118-126.

32. Fras C, Kravetz P, Mody D, Heggeness MH: Substance P-containing nerves within the human vertebral body: An immunohistochemical study of the basivertebral nerve. *Spine J* 2003;3:63-67.

POSTOPERATIVE MANAGEMENT AND REHABILITATION

JUAN M. LATORRE, MD
WILLIAM H. DONOVAN, MD

The thoracolumbar junction is the most commonly injured area of the spine, representing approximately 40% of all spine fractures.[1] A timely and thorough evaluation and rational treatment program are essential for maximizing the patient's neurologic and functional recovery and minimizing associated complications.[2] Serial neurologic evaluations are indicated as well, using the American Spinal Injury Association (ASIA) Impairment Scale.[3]

MANAGEMENT AND REHABILITATION IN THE ABSENCE OF SPINAL CORD INJURY

Controversy persists about the appropriate management of patients with thoracolumbar injuries but no spinal cord injury. Much of the rehabilitation program depends on the approach to treatment, but regardless of the type of treatment, these patients will likely have pain as a limiting factor. Even with surgical instrumentation, some patients have chronic pain following an injury in this area, and of those who do, most report unemployment and permanent disability.[4,5]

Recommendations regarding the orthotic and rehabilitative management for these injuries have changed over time. The early literature advocated a period of bed rest, ranging from 4 to 12 weeks, followed by gradual mobilization.[6-8] Even though a period of bed rest can facilitate bone healing, multiple complications can develop if the patient does not receive meticulous nursing care. The importance of mobilization, as soon as medically and surgically possible, is now recognized. Nonsurgical management of thoracolumbar burst fractures with early casting or bracing and ambulation eliminates prolonged periods of recumbency and hospitalization.[8,9]

Shen and associates[10] recently compared the outcome of surgical treatment with that of nonsurgical treatment in 80 patients (aged 18 to 65 years) with isolated, single-level, neurologically intact burst fractures involving T11 to L2. Patients receiving nonsurgical treatment were allowed activity to the point of pain tolerance using a hyperextension brace beginning on the day the injury occurred. After a follow-up period of 2 years, the authors reported that early activity to the point of pain tolerance could be safely allowed in these patients. In addition, the 2-year satisfaction rate seemed to be lower in patients who received surgical treatment compared with those receiving nonsurgical treatment; one explanation for this result could be that patients in the surgical treatment group may have had higher expectations for recovery.

Compression Fractures

In general, compression fractures of less than 25% are treated with analgesics, immobilization in a thoracic orthotic device, and exclusion from sports participation until evidence of fracture healing exists.[11] Lumbar orthoses function by restricting gross motions of the trunk rather than restricting intervertebral mobility.[12] A more rigid orthosis should be used when rotational control and further reduction of vertebral movement in the sagittal plane are necessary. The two most appropriate forms of bracing for these injuries are the molded thoracolumbar spine orthosis (TLSO) and the Jewett extension orthosis.

In compression fractures of less than 50%, bracing is continued for 6 to 12 weeks, although the duration varies for a variety of factors, including (1) patient response, (2) time to radiologic evidence of fracture healing, (3) persistent pain, and (4) surgeon preference. Compression fractures of more than 50% are associated with a higher incidence of late kyphotic deformity and significant chronic pain.[13] A short period of bed rest followed by mobilization in a TLSO brace and ongoing monitoring for increased kyphosis and neurologic changes are recommended.

Before a rehabilitation program can be initiated, the surgical team should be consulted regarding precautions and/or advice about appropriate exercises. A progressive physical therapy program designed to increase strength and range of motion and restore function while minimizing pain can then be initiated. The duration of therapy required varies; most patients with an uncomplicated initial hospital course are usually discharged with no need for inpatient rehabilitation. In a retrospective review of 27 patients with thoracolumbar fracture but no neurologic deficit or lower extremity fracture, Melchiorre[14] reported that most patients were discharged to their homes with use of a TLSO. A total of 25 (93%) of the patients received physical therapy, and 24 (89%) ambulated independently on discharge after only one or two sessions.

Some patients may report painful spasms; therefore, a short course of an antispasmodic or muscle relaxant may provide some relief. Most pain medications, however, tend to cause constipation. Thus, patients taking these medications should be encouraged to increase their consumption of dietary fiber and to drink plenty of fluids, provided no contraindications exist. A stool softener can also be prescribed. The neurologic status of these patients should be followed closely. Late pain has been reported in as many as 90% of patients, possibly the result of spinal stenosis, segmental instability, foraminal stenosis, or discogenic pain.[15] Bracing may be useful for initial pain control, but it probably does not change the long-term result.

Osteoporotic Fractures

Elderly patients with osteoporotic compression fractures are also often treated with a TLSO and rehabilitation. In patients with well-controlled pain, a less restrictive corset or abdominal binder can be used to facilitate progress in the rehabilitation program. Bracing with a Jewett, cruciform anterior spinal hyperextension (CASH), or chairback brace to maintain the thorax in extension can also be used. Pharmacologic treatment with calcium, vitamin D, estrogens (as indicated), alendronate, raloxifene, and calcitonin is available. Early mobilization is also important to prevent secondary complications of immobility.

Outcomes of Treatment

Patients with thoracolumbar fractures with no neurologic deficit appear to be able to return to work and other activities. Osebold and associates[16] reported on 63 patients with thoracolumbar fractures, most of whom adjusted to their injuries, remaining employed and active. The authors also reported that a detailed, thorough rehabilitation program provided the best functional results and highest patient satisfaction. Andress and associates[17] recently reported that only little more than half of physical laborers who underwent surgical treatment of a similar injury were able to return to their original profession at the time of follow-up. In contrast, 78% of their patients who had a similar injury and treatment but worked in a profession that did not require physical labor were still working in their former jobs. Before the accident, 6% of the overall patient group was permanently disabled or already retired; this percentage increased to 24% at follow-up. Shen and associates[10] also reported that approximately 40% of their patients whose jobs required heavy physical labor before their injury were not able to return to their original jobs.

Return to work and participation in sports after thoracolumbar fractures should be guided by the patient's pain and range of motion, as indicated for specific jobs or sport activities. Radiographic appearance of the fracture often lags behind clinical healing and should not be used as a primary criterion for return to participation. Athletes can return to sports when they regain normal thoracic motion and they are free of pain during activities required by the sport. If repeated direct trauma to the area is likely, the athlete should be padded or wear a protective device.[11]

MANAGEMENT AND REHABILITATION IN PATIENTS WITH A SPINAL CORD INJURY

Assessment and Classification of Spinal Cord Injury

Spinal cord injury has a significant impact on society from the physical, psychosocial, and socioeconomic perspectives. The degree of spinal cord injury is estimated by the extent of neurologic dysfunction based on a comprehensive physical examination. A thorough physical examination is essential in assessing the initial level of injury and is the most accurate method of estimating neurologic recovery[18] (Table 1). After evaluation, injuries can be classified as complete or incomplete spinal cord injury syndromes as discussed in chapter 3 and according to the ASIA Impairment Scale. Reasonable rehabilitation goals and programs can then be established based on the classification of injury.

Initial Rehabilitation

Once patients with a spinal cord injury no longer require intensive care, they should be transferred to a specialized spinal cord injury unit. The initial inpatient rehabilitation is critical to the future health and well-being of the patient. These patients require comprehensive rehabilitation, regardless of the type of initial management of their fractures. Rehabilitation of spinal cord injuries requires systematic care by an experienced multidisciplinary team. Early comprehensive rehabilitation at a specialized spinal cord injury center prevents complications,[19] helps patients attain the highest possible level of function,[20] and provides patients with better overall care.[21] Skillful rehabilitation maximizes the patient's remaining neurologic function and returns most patients to their family and community able to function independently.[22]

Initial priorities include pressure relief for skin, thromboembolism prophylaxis, prevention of gastric ulcers, intermittent catheterization to prevent urine retention, and bowel care to prevent colonic impaction.[19] Patients often have concomitant injuries that may have been missed on initial diagnosis. Awareness and early recognition of potential problems and subsequent intervention for missed injuries will facilitate recovery.

Additional priorities at this time include the following: (1) optimizing nutritional and medical care; (2) maintaining spinal stability to prevent further damage to the spinal cord; (3) diagnosing and treating early complications; (4) preventing joint contractures; (5) ensuring adequate pain management; (6) initiating bowel and bladder management programs; (7) increasing endurance and sitting tolerance; and (8) beginning a comprehensive spinal cord injury education program for the patient, family, and/or caregivers that focuses on functional outcomes, psychological support, and plans for discharge.

Early mobilization is important, and once the spine is stabilized and the patient can tolerate sitting at 60° for approximately 1 hour, more intensive rehabilitation is begun. Mobility and strengthening programs are individualized to each patient's capabilities. Maximizing functional abilities in the following areas is critical: (1) bed mobility; (2) transfers; (3) wheelchair propulsion; (4) self-care skills, including bowel and bladder function and skin care; (5) sexual function; and (6) recreation and community integration.

ASSESSMENT AND MANAGEMENT OF AFFECTED SYSTEMS IN PATIENTS WITH A SPINAL CORD INJURY

Neurologic and Musculoskeletal Systems

Pain

Pain is a common and serious problem in patients with spinal cord injuries and continues to be a significant management problem.[23] The presence of pain and level or completeness of the lesion or type of injury do not appear to be related.[24] New and associates[25] reported that 96% of patients experienced pain, most commonly neuropathic pain or myofascial pain syndrome, at some time during their inpatient rehabilitation. At 1-year follow-up, neuropathic pain remained common whereas myofascial pain syndrome and musculoskeletal pain had decreased.

A history of surgical intervention appears unrelated to pain that persists beyond 2 weeks postoperatively.[26] The reported prevalence of chronic pain has been as high as 94%, but it probably averages 65% of all patients.[27,28] Pain can significantly affect a patient's quality of life and ability to participate in rehabilitation.

Management of spinal cord injury pain remains a clinical challenge because there is no uniformly successful medical or surgical treatment.[29] Different options include

TABLE 1

Lower Extremity Muscle Innervation and Respective Muscle Actions

	L2	L3	L4	L5	S1	S2
Hip flexors	(M) Iliopsoas (S) Rectus femoris (S) Adductor longus	(M) Iliopsoas (M) Rectus femoris (M) Adductor longus	(S) Iliopsoas (m) Tensor fascia lata (M) Rectus femoris (M) Adductor longus	(M) Tensor fascia lata	(S) Tensor fascia lata	
Hip extensors			(m) Semimembran-osus/semitendin-osus	(S) Gluteus maximus (M) Semimembran-osus/semitendin-osus (S) Biceps femoris (long and short heads)	(M) Gluteus maximus (M) Biceps femoris (long and short heads)	(m) Gluteus maximus
Hip abductors			(m) Gluteus medius/minimus (m) Tensor fascia lata	(M) Gluteus medius/minimus (M) Tensor fascia lata	(S) Gluteus medius/minimus (S) Tensor fascia lata	
Hip adductors	(S) Adductor longus	(M) Adductor longus	(M) Adductor longus			
Hip internal rotators			(m) Tensor fascia lata (m) Gluteus minimus	(M) Tensor fascia lata (M) Gluteus minimus	(S) Tensor fascia lata (S) Gluteus minimus	
Hip external rotators				(S) Gluteus maximus	(M) Gluteus maximus	(m) Gluteus maximus
Knee flexors			(m) Semimembran-osus/semitendinosus and biceps femoris (short head)	(M) Semimembran-osus/semitendinosus (S) Biceps femoris (long and short heads)	(M) Biceps femoris (long and short heads) (S) Semimembran-osus/semitendinosus	
Knee extensors	(S) Vastus lateralis/medialis and rectus femoris	(M) Vastus lateralis/medialis and rectus femoris	(M) Vastus lateralis/medialis rectus femoris			
Ankle dorsiflexors			(M) Tibialis anterior.	(M) Tibialis anterior (M) Extensor hallucis	(S) Extensor hallucis	
Ankle plantar flexors				(S) Lateral gastrocnemius	(M) Medial and lateral gastroc-nemius (M) Soleus	(S) Medial gas-trocnemius and soleus
Forefoot evertors				(M) Peroneus group	(S) Peroneus group	
Forefoot invertors				(M) Tibialis posterior (M) Flexor digitorum longus	(S) Tibialis posterior (M) Flexor digitorum longus	
Toe flexors				(M) Flexor digitorum longus	(M) Flexor digitorum longus	
Toe extensors				(M) Extensor hallucis (M) Extensor digitorum brevis (M) Peroneus group	(S) Extensor hallucis (S) Extensor digitorum brevis (S) Peroneus group	

M = Major contribution; S = Sometimes significant contribution; m = Minor contribution

References: AAEM Minimonograph 32: The Electrodiagnostic Examination in Patients with Radiculopathies. MUSCLE and NERVE. December 1998. McPeak L Physiatric History and Examination. In Braddom RL. Physical Medicine and Rehabilitation. Second Edition 2000. 3-45 physical therapy, pharmacologic treatment, behavioral intervention, surgery, or a combination thereof. These treatment options typically provide some isolated pain relief, although complete pain relief often is not possible.[30] The role of psychological, social, and environmental factors must also be considered in the management of these patients.[28,31]

Patients who report neuropathic pain soon after their injury are likely to have chronic pain, which can be severe in some cases. Chronic musculoskeletal pain, in contrast, is more common but less likely to be severe.[32] Patients with chronic pain should be evaluated for associated treatable conditions, such as spinal instability, posttraumatic cystic myelopathy, or an aggravating condition (eg, bladder stone). Pain can also be caused by severe spasticity; drugs that modulate this condition can act as pain relievers.

Diverse treatments can be used to control pain, including noninvasive drug therapies (eg, antidepressants, antiepileptic drugs, and membrane-stabilizing drugs), alternative therapies such as acupuncture,[33] and invasive therapies (eg, nerve blocks, ablative surgery).[34] Gabapentin, a synthetic structural analogue of g-aminobutyric acid (GABA), has been shown to be an effective therapeutic alternative in decreasing neuropathic pain in these patients.[35,36] An initial oral dose of 100 to 300 mg three times a day could be started, with a maximum daily dose of up to 3,600 mg. Botulinum toxin also has been shown to be beneficial in treatment of neuropathic pain disorders. Spinal cord stimulation provides approximately 60% to 80% of long-term pain relief when used in selected patients with spinal cord injuries.[37] Intrathecal clonidine, with or without opioids, may be an effective alternative in the management of intractable spinal cord injury pain and other forms of neuropathic pain.[38] Siddall and associates[39] reported that intrathecal administration of a mixture of clonidine and morphine was more effective than either drug administered alone. Microsurgical approach to the dorsal root entry zone (DREZotomy) in patients with intractable neuropathic pain secondary to spinal cord injury and refractory to nonsurgical management has been reported to provide effective, immediate pain relief in 70% of patients. Approximately 70% of patients with a segmental pain distribution report good results, whereas no patients with predominant infralesional pain report good results.[40]

Spasticity
Spasticity can occur following complete and incomplete cord injuries but usually does not become intense until at least 6 to 12 weeks after injury. It always warrants a careful assessment and management plan. Spasticity in patients with a spinal cord injury frequently does not require treatment. However, it can interfere with positioning, transfers, mobility, and hygiene. Spasticity may also cause pain, loss of range of motion, contractures, sleep disorders, and impaired ambulation in patients with an incomplete lesion.[41] In these patients, preventing nociception and establishing an effective daily stretching and positioning program are the foundations on which all other management plans are based.

Management of spasticity can consist of pharmacotherapy, physiotherapy, and/or surgery.[42] Increased spasticity can be caused by noxious stimuli such as inflammation, urinary tract infection, bladder stones, pressure ulcers, heterotopic ossification, an ingrown toenail, bowel impaction, fractures, or other infections. A correctable cause should be sought and treated. If pharmacologic treatment is selected, baclofen is usually the drug of choice in these patients, although it often is ineffective because of the large dosages required to cross the blood-brain barrier and the potential for subsequent side effects such as hypotonia, sedation/confusion, and withdrawal syndrome. Chronic intrathecal baclofen infusion has been proved to be a safe and effective form of treatment of intractable spasticity in patients with spinal cord injury.[43-45]

Chemical and surgical neurolytic procedures can be used if initial nonsurgical approaches are inadequate. Intramuscular botulinum toxin injections have been used successfully, with effects that generally last for a few months.[46] Patients who receive these injections should also be in a complementary physical therapy program focused on stretching and range of motion. Spinal cord stimulation also appears to be a safe, effective alternative in the management of spasticity in some patients with spinal cord injury.[47] More invasive surgical options, such as tendon lengthening, muscle release, or neurectomy, that have permanent or irreversible consequences are usually best delayed until the spasticity has become static and is severe and intractable to other methods. Central ablative procedures such as rhizotomy and myelotomy are available but are seldom used as alternatives.

Contractures
Contractures are a common, disabling sequelae of spinal cord injury. In addition to controlling spasticity, regular stretching is the principal intervention for the treatment

and prevention of contractures. Serial casting or bracing with progressive joint stretching can be used as well. If nonsurgical management fails, surgery followed by an aggressive rehabilitation program should be considered.

Heterotopic Ossification

Heterotopic ossification (HO) is the development of true bone tissue in soft-tissue planes surrounding a joint. It is a frequent complication following spinal cord injury, with an incidence of up to 30%. Up to 10% of those affected have severe functional limitations.[48] HO develops in the proximal joints below the level of the injury, most commonly in patients with complete lower cervical or thoracic lesions. Heterotopic bone formation is more likely to develop in patients with spasticity than in patients with flaccid muscles.[49,50] HO is most frequently detected 1 to 3 months after spinal cord injury.[51] The etiology is unknown.

Presenting signs and symptoms can include a combination of loss of hip range of motion, elevated serum alkaline phosphatase level, fever, generalized or localized lower extremity swelling, erythema, and occasional joint tenderness. This constellation of findings can make HO difficult to distinguish from cellulitis, osteomyelitis, hematoma, or thrombophlebitis. HO can result in significantly limited range of motion or nerve entrapments, but most often it is an incidental subclinical finding. Elevated serum alkaline phosphatase levels and a positive bone scan, in addition to restricted range of motion, are usually indicative of HO.[52]

Optimal management consists of a combination of range-of-motion exercises, diphosphonates, nonsteroidal anti-inflammatory drugs, radiation therapy, and in some cases, surgical resection. Orzel and Rudd[52] and Silver[53] found that vigorous range-of-motion exercises in the acute stage actually aggravated the clinical picture and increased the amount of HO in most of their patients. It also diminished joint mobility in the long term and prolonged the period of rehabilitation. Thus, gentle range-of-motion and stretching programs are probably safe to maintain range of motion while preventing additional HO formation. Aggressive stretching and range of motion should not be resumed until the acute inflammation subsides.

Diphosphonates are frequently used, although routine prophylaxis has not been proved to be effective.[49] Etidronate is a common drug of choice, usually an oral dose of 20 mg/kg/d for 2 weeks, followed by 10 mg/kg/d for at least 10 weeks. An intravenous preparation of etidronate also is available for acute use. Indomethacin should be considered as an adjunct or alternative to other existing therapies.[54] Banovac and associates[55] conducted a randomized, controlled trial to evaluate the effectiveness of indomethacin in preventing HO following spinal cord injury. The authors reported that slow-release indomethacin, in a dose of 75 mg daily during the first 2 months after spinal cord injury, is effective in preventing HO in a significant number of patients. In patients in whom HO continues to develop despite pharmacologic treatment, radiation therapy can be a safe and effective local treatment option.[56]

Surgical resection is generally reserved for situations in which (1) nonsurgical management has failed, (2) the patient has severely limited range of motion that interferes with function, or (3) the development of a pressure ulcer is a concern. The possibility of recurrence following surgery may be limited by use of medications and irradiation.[56] Osteonecrosis of the femoral head after combination treatment of surgery, irradiation, and a nonsteroidal anti-inflammatory drug has been reported.[57]

Osteopenia and Osteoporosis

Another common problem in patients with a spinal cord injury is the development of osteopenia below the level of the injury. The characteristic bone loss can be substantial in the lower extremities, equaling approximately 50% of normal values in the proximal tibia, the result of which has been a high incidence of low-impact fractures.[58] Treatment with intravenous pamidronate and ability to ambulate within the first 6 months after acute spinal cord injury prevents bone density loss.[59] An intensive exercise regimen has not been shown to prevent demineralization in the lower extremities, although such a regimen may help preserve arm bone mass in male patients with a spinal cord injury.[60]

Cardiovascular System

Patients with a spinal cord injury are more susceptible to cardiac morbidity and mortality soon after their injury. Cardiovascular disease is becoming a leading cause of mortality in this patient population; therefore, modification of risk factors is more important,[61] as is fitness training.[62,63] Spinal cord injury alone does not promote atherosclerosis. However, in association with multiple secondary comorbidities, patients are predisposed to relatively greater risk of heart disease.

Deep venous thrombosis (DVT) and pulmonary embolism are common complications of acute spinal cord injury. DVT is potentially dangerous, and its prevention represents a major challenge. Duplex ultrasound is an important noninvasive technique to screen these patients for DVT on admission to a rehabilitation setting, regardless of the completeness, level, or cause of injury.[64]

The high rate of DVT in this population has led to numerous studies to identify the most effective regimens of prophylaxis. Pneumatic compression devices can be used for the first 2 weeks, followed by use of compression hose. Benefit from sequential compression devices continues to 6 weeks after injury.[65] When thromboprophylaxis has been delayed for more than 72 hours after injury, tests to exclude the presence of leg thrombi should be performed before applying compression devices. Sequential compression devices provide adequate DVT prophylaxis with a low failure rate (3% to 8%) and no device-related complications. Foot pumps appear to be a reasonable alternative when lower extremity fractures preclude use of these devices.[66] The effectiveness of sequential compression devices may be enhanced by combined use with other antithrombotic agents.

Prophylaxis with low molecular weight heparin and elastic stockings significantly reduces the frequency of DVT during initial rehabilitation.[67] The Consortium for Spinal Cord Injury Medicine Clinical Practice Guidelines[68] recommends anticoagulant prophylaxis with either low molecular weight heparin or adjusted-dose unfractioned heparin to be initiated within 72 hours after spinal cord injury, provided there is no acute bleeding or coagulopathy. Anticoagulants should be continued for 8 weeks in patients with incomplete motor or uncomplicated complete injuries and for 12 weeks in patients with complete motor injury and other risk factors (eg, lower extremity fractures, a history of thrombosis, cancer, heart failure, obesity, or age over 70 years). Unless contraindicated, this recommendation also applies to patients with inferior vena cava filters in place because their risk for DVT equals that of patients without the filter. In fact, patients with filters may be at greater risk for recurrence.[69] In patients with multiple risk factors, placement of an inferior vena cava filter should be considered.[70]

Pulmonary System

Atelectasis and pneumonia are the most common pulmonary complications following acute spinal cord injury, although they are much less frequently associated with thoracolumbar injuries than with injuries higher in the spine. Pulmonary embolism can occur, sometimes with serious consequences, in these patients, but in our experience it rarely causes pulmonary infarction if detected and treated promptly. Patients with concurrent chest and/or lung trauma require precautions against pneumonia, and ventilator support may be needed for the short term.

Genitourinary System

Initial bladder management for patients with a spinal cord injury usually consists of insertion of an indwelling catheter, as the bladder is likely to be flaccid during the initial period of spinal shock. The catheter should be left in place until the patient no longer requires IV fluids or nasogastric nutritional supplementation. An intermittent catheterization program should then be implemented.[71] Catheterization is performed every 4 to 6 hours, with a goal of maintaining output below 400 to 500 mL.

Biering-Sorensen[72] reported that urinary tract infection continues to be the most frequently reported secondary impairment in patients with spinal cord lesion. The author showed that the most prevalent risk indicator for urinary tract infection was the presence of an dwelling catheter. Prophylaxis is not considered an effective strategy for preventing recurrent urinary tract infections. Rather, it is better to treat the recurrent infections than to maintain the patient on an antimicrobial so that resistant bacteria will not develop.

Urodynamic evaluation is recommended for all patients with a spinal cord injury, with the initial urodynamics study done after following the spinal shock phase.[73] Treatment should be guided by these urodynamic data.[73,74] With appropriate surveillance and management, morbidity and mortality from neurogenic bladder dysfunction can be successfully prevented.[75] Razdan and associates[76] recently reported that most physicians (85%) favor a yearly renal ultrasound for routine surveillance of the upper urinary tracts, whereas more than half (65%) routinely use videourodynamic studies for evaluation of the lower urinary tract. They also reported that the combination of clean intermittent catheterization plus anticholinergic agents is the favored management of a hyperreflexic bladder, whereas clean intermittent catheterization alone is preferred for an areflexic bladder.

Gastrointestinal System

Spinal cord injury has a significant effect on normal bowel function. During the first 3 weeks of hospitalization, gastrointestinal complications develop in about 6% of patients; the most common disorders are ileus, peptic ulcer disease, and gastritis.[77] Neurogenic colonic dysfunction is a particularly distressing and limiting impairment for a substantial proportion of these patients, has a significant impact on quality of life, and is a cause of morbidity and death.[78] Initial evaluation to identify upper and/or lower motor neuron dysfunction is indicated. Bowel management is also required to promote evacuation and prevent chronic constipation and should be implemented after the ileus is resolved and the patient's diet (oral or nasogastric) has been resumed. An optimal bowel program should (1) achieve effective, efficient evacuation in a predictable and socially acceptable time, (2) avoid short- and long-term complications, and (3) eliminate inadequate intestinal evacuation habits.[79] Stool softeners (100 mg oral docusate sodium twice daily), bowel stimulants (two senna tablets daily), and/or pre-mixed commercial preparations (two tablets daily) are often integral to an optimal bowel management program. These tablets typically are taken 8 hours before planned bowel evacuation. Enemas can be used as needed.

Integumentary System

Pressure ulcers remain a prevalent health problem for patients with a spinal cord injury. Pressure ulceration can confine an otherwise independent individual to bed rest. In patients with chronic spinal cord injury, the annual incidence is nearly 25%.[80] The prevalence of pressure ulcers appears to be higher with complete neurologic lesions than with incomplete lesions,[81] and the risk for skin breakdown is higher with paraplegia than with tetraplegia.[82] Pressure ulcers usually develop at bony prominences as a result of four etiologic elements: pressure, shearing forces, friction, and moisture.[83] The most commonly affected sites are the sacrum, ischium, trochanters, and ankles and heels.[84] In the acute setting, a proper mattress, meticulous nursing care, and frequent position changes are critical.

The best treatment of pressure ulcers is prevention. Preventive strategies include decreasing the effects of pressure by choosing an optimal cushioning surface (mattress and wheelchair cushion) to evenly distribute pressure in different areas while decreasing it on bony surfaces, assessing nutritional status, avoiding excessive bed rest, frequently changing bed position, providing pressure relief maneuvers when in the wheelchair, and preserving skin integrity. Once a pressure ulcer develops,

an initial assessment, including staging the ulcer, is required. Treatment principles include reducing local pressure, friction, and shear forces; optimizing wound care; cleaning and removing necrotic debris; managing bacterial contamination; and correcting and treating factors that retard wound healing such as nutritional deficits.[83,85] Cruse and associates[86] reported that patients with pressure ulcers may have decreased serum levels of prealbumin and zinc. In addition to routine comprehensive nutritional support, vitamin A and zinc (when zinc levels are low) should be added to the nutritional support.[87] For deep wounds, a vacuum-assisted closure system is useful.[88] For superficial necrotic wounds, enzymatic therapy can enhance débridement. For clean wounds, growth factors such as becaplermin topical can promote healing. Surgery is a last resort because of the high rate of complications; however, it can be very effective in restoring functional positioning.[89]

Social and Psychological Systems

While the psychological and societal consequences of spinal cord injury can be devastating, quality of life has been found to be acceptable in most long-term survivors. Quality of life is less influenced by the neurologic status than by the degree to which the patient can resume his or her role in society.[90] In general, patients with a spinal cord injury at the thoracolumbar level should be able to (1) return to most jobs, with necessary workplace modifications; (2) drive with or without hand controls, depending upon lower extremity residual function; and (3) achieve an excellent degree of autonomy. Employment rates decline immediately following a spinal cord injury but increase subsequently, though not to the level of the general population. Those who have a job and those who can drive are generally younger, autonomous, and have a higher quality of life.[91] This fact stresses the importance of providing these patient with vocational and driving rehabilitation.

Psychiatric assessment is warranted for patients with signs of depression or unresolved adjustment disorder. Suicide rates are higher in this population than in the general population and higher among paraplegics than in tetraplegics.[92]

Neurologic Prognosis

A comprehensive physical examination is essential to identify the initial level and classification of the injury and is the most accurate way to predict neurologic recovery.[93] Within 72 hours to 1 month after a spinal cord injury, it is possible to predict with reasonable accuracy the magnitude of expected recovery based on physical examination.[94] The preservation of pinprick sensation in a motor segment with grade 0 power indicates an 85% chance of motor recovery to at least grade 3.[95] Catz and associates[96] evaluated 250 patients with a traumatic spinal cord lesion. During rehabilitation, 27% of all patients who were Frankel grades A, B, or C on admission, and 54% of those who were grade C, experienced full or substantial neurologic recovery (grade D or E). Other diagnostic tests, including somatosensory evoked potentials, MRI, and transcranial magnetic stimulation, may be helpful in further predicting outcome when used in association with the clinical examination, but these tests are often superfluous.

Understanding neurologic recovery should help predict ultimate functional capability and potential home needs.[93] Patients with an initial incomplete injury to the cord or cauda equina are thought to have a better chance of neurologic improvement than patients who initially have a complete cord injury.[97] In patients with incomplete spinal trauma, significant changes in neurologic function may continue for years.[98]

Significant efforts have been made to estimate the prognosis and recovery for ambulation in patients with a spinal cord injury. Patients with a motor incomplete spinal cord injury (ie, those with any voluntary muscle function more than three myotomes below the motor level) who recover more than 3/5 quadriceps strength within 2 months of the injury have an excellent prognosis for subsequent ambulation within 6 months.[99] In a study of 98 consecutive patients with neurologic impairment following a thoracolumbar injury, Lifeso and associates[100] reported that all patients with incomplete paraplegia (nine patients) regained the ability to walk. Three of the 12 patients with complete paraplegia improved sufficiently to walk with bilateral ankle-foot orthoses.

Outcomes and Functional Expectations

The Functional Independence Measure (FIM) has emerged as a standard assessment instrument for use in rehabilitation and therapy programs for disabled persons, including those with spinal cord injury.[101] The FIM uses a seven-point scale to measure 18 different items in six different categories, including self-care, bowel and bladder continence, mobility, locomotion, communication, and social cognition. Motor items appear to accurately represent the functional status of individuals, and FIM motor scores can illustrate improvements in neurologic status and ASIA scores.

The expected outcomes of patients with a thoracolumbar spinal cord injury depend on the precise level and the degree of injury. Patients with an injury at the T10-L1 level should be independent in all their functional transfers and wheelchair mobility; they can also potentially stand with braces for limited exercise. Household ambulation is possible for these patients with knee-ankle-foot orthoses and crutches or a walker but requires an extreme amount of energy and motivation. Independence in all self-care activities is expected. These patients usually require some assistance with heavy housekeeping, typically about 2 hours of assistance daily. A patient injured at the L2–L3 level will have full, or at least partial, use of the iliopsoas and the quadriceps; both are key muscles in the gait cycle. Generally, the minimum requirement for a patient to achieve community ambulation is a high degree of motivation and at least L2 motor function (ie, hip flexion) on one side and L3 motor function (ie, knee extension and hip flexion) on the other side (Table 1). At this level, orthotic assistance of a knee-ankle-foot orthosis and an ankle-foot orthosis, along with a walker, cane, and/or crutches is necessary. This gait may be sufficient for short community ambulation but still is laborious, and some patients may prefer a wheelchair.

SUMMARY AND CONCLUSIONS

Spinal cord injuries can have a profound impact on the physical, emotional, vocational, and social aspects of a person's life. The sudden and often dramatic changes resulting from a spinal cord injury require a comprehensive rehabilitation program to maximize the patient's progress toward adapting to changes in independent functioning and returning to leading a productive life at home, school, work, and in the community.

REFERENCES

1. Holmes JF, Miller PQ, Panacek EA, Lin S, Horne NS, Mower WR: Epidemiology of thoracolumbar spine injury in blunt trauma. *Acad Emerg Med* 2001;8:866-872.
2. Spivak JM, Vaccaro AR, Cotler JM: Thoracolumbar spine trauma: I. Evaluation and classification. *J Am Acad Orthop Surg* 1995;3:345-352.
3. American Spinal Cord Injury Association: *Standards for Neurological and Functional Classification of Spinal Cord Injury, Revised*. Atlanta, GA, American Spinal Cord Injury Association, 2002.

4. Knop C, Fabian HF, Bastian L, Blauth M: Late results of thoracolumbar fractures after posterior instrumentation and transpedicular bone grafting. *Spine* 2001;26:88-99.

5. Sanderson PL, Fraser RD, Hall DJ, Cain CM, Osti OL, Potter GR: Short segment fixation of thoracolumbar burst fractures without fusion. *Eur Spine J* 1999;8:495-500.

6. Davies WE, Morris JH, Hill V: An analysis of conservative (non-surgical) management of TL fractures and fracture-dislocations with neural damage. *J Bone Joint Surg Am* 1980;62:1324-1328.

7. Jacobs RR, Asher MA, Snider RK: Thoracolumbar spinal injuries, a comparative study of recumbent and operative treatment in 100 patients. *Spine* 1980;5:463-477.

8. Krompinger WJ, Fredrickson BE, Mino DE, Hanson AY: Conservative treatment of fractures of the thoracic and lumbar spine. *Orthop Clin North Am* 1986;17:161-170.

9. Cantor JB, Lebwohl NH, Garvey T, Eismont FJ: Nonoperative management of stable thoracolumbar burst fractures with early ambulation and bracing. *Spine* 1993;18:971-976.

10. Shen WJ, Liu TJ, Shen Y: Nonoperative treatment versus posterior fixation for thoracolumbar junction burst fractures without neurologic deficit. *Spine* 2001;26:1038-1045.

11. Eismont FJ, Kitchel SH, DeLee JC: Thoracolumbar spine: Section A. Thoracolumbar spine in the adult, in *DeLee and Drez's Orthopaedic Sports Medicine: Principles and Practice*, ed 2. Philadelphia, PA, WB Saunders, 2003, vol 2, pp 1525-1561.

12. Axelsson P, Johnson R, Stromqvist B: Effect of lumbar orthosis on intervertebral mobility: A roentgen stereophotogrammetric analysis. *Spine* 1992;17:678-681.

13. Holdsworth F: Fractures, dislocations and fracture-dislocations of the spine. *J Bone Joint Surg Am* 1970;52:1534-1551.

14. Melchiorre PJ: Acute hospitalization and discharge outcome of neurologically intact trauma patients sustaining thoracolumbar vertebral fractures managed conservatively with thoracolumbosacral orthoses and physical therapy. *Arch Phys Med Rehabil* 1999;80:221-224.

15. Jodoin A, Dupuis P, Fraser M: Unstable fractures of the thoracolumbar spine. A 10 year experience at Sacre-Coeur Hospital. *J Trauma* 1985;25:197-202.

16. Osebold WR, Weinstein SL, Sprague BL: Thoracolumbar spine fractures. Results of treatment. *Spine* 1981;6:13-34.

17. Andress H, Braun H, Helmberger T, Schürmann M, Hertlein H, Hartl WH: Long-term results after posterior fixation of thoraco-lumbar burst fractures. *Injury* 2002;33:357-365.

18. Kirshblum SC, O'Connor KC: Levels of spinal cord injury and predictors of neurologic recovery. *Phys Med Rehabil Clin N Am* 2000;11:1-27.

19. Kirshblum SC, Groah SL, McKinley WO, Gittler MS: Spinal cord injury medicine: 1. Etiology, classification, and acute medical management. *Arch Phys Med Rehabil* 2002;83:S50-S57, S90-S98.

20. Sonntag V, Douglas R: Management of spinal cord trauma. *Neurosurg Clin N Am* 1990;1:729-750.

21. Smith M: Efficacy of specialist versus non-specialist management of spinal cord injury within the UK. *Spinal Cord* 2002;40:10-16.

22. Woolsey RM: Modern concepts of therapy and management of spinal cord injuries. *Crit Rev Neurobiol* 1988;4:137-156.

23. Finnerup NB, Johannesen IL, Sindrup SH, Bach FW, Jensen TS: Pain and dysesthesia in patients with spinal cord injury: A postal survey. *Spinal Cord* 2001;39:256-262.

24. Siddall PJ, Taylor DA, McClelland JM, Rutkowski SB, Cousins MJ: Pain report and the relationship of pain to physical factors in the first 6 months following spinal cord injury. *Pain* 1999;81:187-197.

25. New PW, Lim TC, Hill ST, Brown DJ: A survey of pain during rehabilitation after acute spinal cord injury. *Spinal Cord* 1997;35:658-663.

26. Sved P, Siddall PJ, McClelland J, Cousins MJ: Relationship between surgery and pain following spinal cord injury. *Spinal Cord* 1997;35:526-530.

27. Botterell EH, Callaghan JC, Jousse T: Pain in paraplegia; clinical management and surgical treatment. *Proc R Soc Med* 1954;47:281-288.

28. Siddall PJ, Loeser JD: Pain following spinal cord injury. *Spinal Cord* 2001;39:63-73.

29. Burchiel KJ, Hsu FP: Pain and spasticity after spinal cord injury: Mechanisms and treatment. *Spine* (24 Suppl) 2001;26:146-160.

30. Bryce TN, Ragnarsson KT: Pain after spinal cord injury. *Phys Med Rehabil Clin N Am* 2000;11:157-168.

31. Richards JS, Meredith RL, Nepomuceno C: Psycho-social aspects of chronic pain in spinal cord injury. *Pain* 1980;8:355-366.

32. Siddall PJ, McClelland JM, Rutkowski SB, Cousins MJ: A longitudinal study of the prevalence and characteristics of pain in the first 5 years following spinal cord injury. *Pain* 2003;103:249-257.

33. Rapson LM, Wells N, Pepper J, Majid N, Boon H: Acupuncture as a promising treatment for below-level central neuropathic pain: A retrospective study. *J Spinal Cord Med* 2003;26:21-26.

34. Chong MS, Bajwa ZH: Diagnosis and treatment of neuropathic pain. *J Pain Symptom Manage* 2003;25:S4-S11.

35. Ahn SH, Park HW, Lee BS, et al: Gabapentin effect on neuropathic pain compared among patients with spinal cord injury and different durations of symptoms. *Spine* 2003;28:341-346.

36. To TP, Lim TC, Hill ST, et al: Gabapentin for neuropathic pain following spinal cord injury. *Spinal Cord* 2002;40:282-285.

37. Krames E: Implantable devices for pain control: Spinal cord stimulation and intrathecal therapies. *Best Pract Res Clin Anaesthesiol* 2002;16:619-649.

38. Siddall PJ, Gray M, Rutkowski S, Cousins MJ: Intrathecal morphine and clonidine in the management of spinal cord injury pain: a case report. *Pain* 1994;59:147-148.

39. Siddall PJ, Molloy AR, Walker S, Mather LE, Rutkowski SB: The efficacy of intrathecal morphine and clonidine in the treatment of pain after SCI. *Anesth Analg* 2000;91:1493-1498.

40. Sindou M, Mertens P, Wael M: Microsurgical DREZotomy for pain due to spinal cord and/or cauda equina injuries: Long-term results in a series of 44 patients. *Pain* 2001;92:159-171.

41. Taricco M, Adone R, Pagliacci C, Telaro E: Pharmacological interventions for spasticity following spinal cord injury. *Cochrane Library* 2000;1.

42. Eltorai I, Montroy R: Muscle release in the management of spasticity in spinal cord injury. *Paraplegia* 1990;28:433-440.

43. Korenkov AI, Niendorf WR, Darwish N, Glaeser E, Gaab MR: Continuous intrathecal infusion of baclofen in patients with spasticity caused by SCI. *Neurosurg Rev* 2002;25:228-230.

44. Akman MN, Loubser PG, Donovan WH, O'Neill ME, Rossi CD: Intrathecal baclofen: Does tolerance occur? *Paraplegia* 1993;31:516-520.

45. Penn RD, Savoy SM, Corcos D, et al: Intrathecal baclofen for severe spinal spasticity. *N Engl J Med* 1989;320:1517-1521.

46. Yablon SA: Botulinum neurotoxin intramuscular chemodenervation. Role in the management of spastic hypertonia and related motor disorders. *Phys Med Rehabil Clin N Am* 2001;12:833-874.

47. Barolat G, Singh-Sahni K, Staas WE Jr, Shatin D, Ketcik B, Allen K: Epidural spinal cord stimulation in the management of spasms in spinal cord injury: A prospective study. *Stereotact Funct Neurosurg* 1995;64:153-164.

48. Subbarao JV, Garrison SJ: Heterotopic ossification: Diagnosis and management, current concepts and controversies. *J Spinal Cord Med* 1999;22:273-283.

49. Dai L: Heterotopic ossification of the hip after spinal cord injury. *Chin Med J (Engl)*. 1998;111:1099-1101.

50. van Kuijk AA, Geurts ACH, van Kuppevelt HJM: Neurogenic heterotopic ossification in spinal cord injury. *Spinal Cord* 2002;40:313-326.

51. Garland DE: A clinical perspective on common forms of acquired heterotopic ossification. *Clin Orthop* 1991;263:13-29.

52. Orzel JA, Rudd TG: Heterotopic bone formation: Clinical, laboratory and imaging correlation. *J Nucl Med* 1985;26:125-132.

53. Silver J: Comment on "Neurogenic heterotopic ossification in spinal cord injury" article. *Spinal Cord* 2003;41:421-422.

54. Schurch B, Capaul M, Vallotton MB, Rossier AB: Prostaglandin E2 measurements: Their value in the early diagnosis of heterotopic ossification in spinal cord injury patients. *Arch Phys Med Rehabil* 1997;78:687-691.

55. Banovac K, Williams JM, Patrick LD, Haniff YM: Prevention of heterotopic ossification after spinal cord injury with indomethacin. *Spinal Cord* 2001;39:370-374.

56. Sautter-Bihl ML, Liebermeister E, Nanassy A: Radiotherapy as a local treatment option for heterotopic ossifications in patients with spinal cord injury. *Spinal Cord* 2000;38:33-36.

57. van Kuijk AA, van Kuppevelt HJ, van der Schaaf DB: Osteonecrosis after treatment for heterotopic ossification in spinal cord injury with the combination of surgery, irradiation, and an NSAID. *Spinal Cord* 2000;38:319-324.

58. Mohr T, Podenphant J, Biering-Sorensen F, Galbo H, Thamsborg G, Kjaer M: Increased bone mineral density after prolonged electrically induced cycle training of paralyzed limbs in spinal cord injured man. *Calcif Tissue Int* 1997;61:22-25.

59. Nance PW, Schryvers O, Leslie W, Ludwig S, Krahn J: Intravenous pamidronate attenuates bone density loss after acute spinal cord injury. *Arch Phys Med Rehabil* 1999;80:243-251.

60. Jones LM, Legge M, Goulding A: Intensive exercise may preserve bone mass of the upper limbs in spinal cord injured males but does not retard demineralisation of the lower body. *Spinal Cord* 2002;40:230-235.

61. Groah SL, Stiens SA, Gittler MS, Kirshblum SC, McKinley WO: Spinal cord injury medicine: 5. Preserving wellness and independence of the aging patient with SCI: A primary care approach for the rehabilitation medicine specialist. *Arch Phys Med Rehabil* 2002;83 (3 suppl 1):S82-S89, S90-S98.

62. Phillips WT: Effect of spinal cord injury on the heart and cardiovascular fitness. *Curr Probl Cardiol* 1998;23:641-716.

63. Nash MS, Jacobs PL, Mendez AJ, Goldberg RB: Circuit resistance training improves the atherogenic lipid profiles of persons with chronic paraplegia. *J Spinal Cord Med* 2001;24:2-9.

64. Powell M, Kirshblum S, O'Connor KC: Duplex ultrasound screening for deep vein thrombosis in SCI patients at rehabilitation admission. *Arch Phys Med Rehabil* 1999;80:1044-1046.

65. Winemiller MH, Stolp-Smith KA, Silverstein MD, Therneau TM: Prevention of venous thromboembolism in patients with spinal cord injury: Effects of sequential pneumatic compression and heparin. *J Spinal Cord Med* 1999;22:182-191.

66. Spain DA, Bergamini TM, Hoffmann JF, Carrillo EH, Richardson JD: Comparison of sequential compression devices and foot pumps for prophylaxis of deep venous thrombosis in high-risk trauma patients. *Am Surg* 1998;64:522-526.

67. Riklin C, Baumberger M, Wick L, Michel D, Sauter B, Knecht H: Deep vein thrombosis and heterotopic ossification in spinal cord injury: A 3 year experience at the Swiss Paraplegic Centre Nottwil. *Spinal Cord* 2003;41:192-198.

68. Consortium for Spinal Cord Medicine: *Prevention of Thromboembolism in Spinal Cord Injury*, ed 2. Washington, DC, Paralyzed Veterans of America, 1999.

69. Green D, Hull RD, Mammen EF, Merli GJ, Weingarden SI, Yao JS: Deep vein thrombosis in spinal cord injury. Summary and recommendations. *Chest* 1992;102(suppl 6):633S-635S.

70. Maxwell RA, Chavarria-Aguilar M, Cockerham WT, et al: Routine prophylactic vena cava filtration is not indicated after acute spinal cord injury. *J Trauma* 2002;52:902-906.

71. Binard JE, Persky L, Lockhart JL, Kelley B: Intermittent catheterization the right way! (Volume vs. time-directed). *J Spinal Cord Med* 1996;19:194-196.

72. Biering-Sorensen F: Urinary tract infection in individuals with spinal cord lesion. *Curr Opin Urol* 2002;12:45-49.

73. Nygaard IE, Kreder KJ: Spine update: Urological management in patients with spinal cord injuries. *Spine* 1996;21:128-132.

74. Jamil F: Towards a catheter free status in neurogenic bladder dysfunction: A review of bladder management options in spinal cord injury (SCI). *Spinal Cord* 2001;39:355-361.

75. Burns AS, Rivas DA, Ditunno JF: The management of neurogenic bladder and sexual dysfunction after spinal cord injury. *Spine* 2001;26(suppl 24): S129-S136.

76. Razdan S, Leboeuf L, Meinbach DS, Weinstein D, Gousse AE: Current practice patterns in the urologic surveillance and management of patients with SCI. *Urology* 2003;61:893-896.

77. Albert TJ, Levine MJ, Balderston RA, Cotler JM: Gastrointestinal complications in spinal cord injury. *Spine* 1991;16:S522-S525.

78. Chen D, Nussbaum SB: The gastrointestinal system and bowel management following spinal cord injury. *Phys Med Rehabil Clin N Am* 2000;11:45-56.

79. Correa GI, Rotter KP: Clinical evaluation and management of neurogenic bowel after spinal cord injury. *Spinal Cord* 2000;38:301-308.

80. Whiteneck GG, Charlifue SW, Frankel HL, et al: Mortality, morbidity, and psychosocial out-comes of persons spinal cord injured more than 20 years ago. *Paraplegia* 1992;30:617-630.

81. Richardson RR, Meyer PR: Prevalence and incidence of pressure sores in acute spinal cord injuries. *Paraplegia* 1981;19:235-247.

82. Byrne DW, Salzberg CA: Major risk factors for pressure ulcers in the spinal cord disabled: A literature review. *Spinal Cord* 1996;34:255-263.

83. Longe RL: Current concepts in clinical therapeutics: Pressure sores. *Clin Pharm* 1986;5:669-681.

84. Yarkony GM: Pressure ulcers: A review. *Arch Phys Med Rehabil* 1994;75:908-917.

85. Thomas DR: Prevention and treatment of pressure ulcers: What works? What doesn't? *Cleve Clin J Med* 2001;68:704-707, 710-714, 717-722.

86. Cruse JM, Lewis RE, Roe DL, et al: Facilitation of immune function, healing of pressure ulcers, and nutritional status in spinal cord injury patients. *Exp Mol Pathol* 2000;68:38-54.

87. Singer P: Nutritional care to prevent and heal pressure ulcers. *Isr Med Assoc J* 2002;4:713-716.

88. Morykwas MJ, Argenta LC, Shelton-Brown EI, et al: Vacuum-assisted closure: A new method for wound control and treatment: Animal studies and basic foundation. *Ann Plast Surg* 1997;38:553-562.

89. Netscher D, Clamon J, Fincher L, Thompson R: Surgical repair of pressure ulcers. *Plast Surg Nurs* 1996;16:225-233, 239.

90. Manns PJ, Chad KE: Components of quality of life for persons with a quadriplegic and paraplegic spinal cord injury. *Qual Health Res* 2001;11:795-811.

91. Franceschini M, Di Clemente B, Rampello A, Nora M, Spizzichino L: Longitudinal outcome 6 years after spinal cord injury. *Spinal Cord* 2003;41:280-285.

92. Hartkopp A, Bronnum-Hansen H, Seidenschnur AM, Biering-Sorensen F: Suicide in a spinal cord injured population: Its relation to functional status. *Arch Phys Med Rehabil* 1998;79:1356-1361.

93. Kirshblum SC, O'Connor KC: Predicting neurologic recovery in traumatic cervical spinal cord injury. *Arch Phys Med Rehabil* 1998;79:1456-1466.

94. Burns AS, Ditunno JF: Establishing prognosis and maximizing functional outcomes after spinal cord injury: A review of current and future directions in rehabilitation management. *Spine* 2001;26:S137-S145.

95. Poynton AR, O'Farrell DA, Shannon F, Murray P, McManus F, Walsh MG: Sparing of sensation to pin prick predicts recovery of a motor segment after injury to the spinal cord. *J Bone Joint Surg Br* 1997;79:952-954.

96. Catz A, Thaleisnik M, Fishel B, et al: Recovery of neurologic function after spinal cord injury in Israel. *Spine* 2002;27:1733-1735.

97. Kim NH, Lee HM, Chan IM: Neurologic injury and recovery in patients with burst fractures of the thoracolumbar spine. *Spine* 1999;24:290-294.

98. Piepmeier JM, Jenkins NR: Late neurological changes following traumatic spinal cord injury. *J Neurosurg* 1988;69:399-402.

99. Crozier KS, Cheng LL, Graziani V, Zorn G, Herbison G, Ditunno JF: Spinal cord injury: Prognosis for ambulation based on quadriceps recovery. *Paraplegia* 1992;30:762-767.

100. Lifeso RM, Arabie KM, Kadhi SK: Fractures of the thoraco-lumbar spine. *Paraplegia* 1985;23:207-224.

101. Grey N, Kennedy P: The Functional Independence Measure: A comparative study of clinician and self ratings. *Paraplegia* 1993;31:457-461.

CHAPTER 13

COMPLICATIONS

CHARLES A. REITMAN, MD

The incidence of complications is particularly high for thoracolumbar injuries, regardless of whether the patient is managed nonsurgically or surgically, because of the character of these injuries, the high rate of associated injuries, and the nature of spinal surgery. Knop and associates[1] reviewed 682 thoracolumbar fractures treated surgically and found the rate of intraoperative complications alone was 15%. In addition, several complications that are nonspinal in origin are well recognized to be commonly associated with thoracolumbar injuries. Many of the complications encountered in the management of these injuries are summarized in Table 1.

NONSURGICAL COMPLICATIONS

Neurologic Deficits

Possibly the biggest initial concern with thoracolumbar injuries is the potential for a neurologic deficit. Any initial deficit is related to the injury itself and to the amount of displacement at the time of injury. The severity of the damage caused by this dynamic mechanism is not always reflected in the static imaging studies obtained in the emergency department. Proper initial provisional immobilization is required to optimize the final neurologic condition because improper immobilization can result in progression of the deficit. Secondary injury mechanisms, such as an expanding epidural hematoma, may play a role.

Therefore, a progressive neurologic deficit needs to be diagnosed immediately and managed with prompt surgical decompression and stabilization. To expedite this decision making, frequent and accurate serial examinations must be performed, beginning with prompt evaluation in the emergency department.

Late onset of increasing neurologic deficits can also arise secondary to the development of a syrinx. The neurologic decline can be progressive; therefore, a high index of suspicion should be maintained. The diagnosis usually can be confirmed with MRI. Surgical management involves shunting of the syrinx.

Dural Tears

Dural tears can occur with thoracolumbar injuries. In addition to being associated with spinal cord transection, dural tears are most commonly reported in the presence of a burst fracture with concurrent laminar fracture. Unlike dural tears associated with cerebrospinal fluid leakage following elective surgery, which can lead to spinal headaches or durocutaneous fistulas, with dural tears associated with thoracolumbar fractures the major concern is impingement of nerve roots in the posterior fracture that may result in a neurologic deficit.[2,3] Failure to release entrapped nerve roots and repair the dura could limit the potential for neurologic recovery. This problem is more commonly seen in the lumbar spine than in the thoracic spine. Therefore, in any patient with a burst injury and laminar fracture that requires surgery, posterior exploration to assess for dural continuity and

Complications Associated With Thoracolumbar Injuries

Infection
Pain
Blood loss
Technical—acute
  Hardware malposition
  Inadequate decompression
  Wrong-site surgery
  Improper reduction
Technical—delayed
  Deformity/loss of correction of alignment
  Hardware failure
  Pseudarthrosis
Neurologic
  Increased neurologic deficit
  Sympathectomy
Visceral
  Pulmonary complications
  Bowel function
  Ureter injuries
  Thoracic duct lacerations
Vascular injuries
Bone graft site problems

possible nerve root entrapment should be considered before stabilization. In patients exhibiting a neurologic deficit with this fracture pattern, posterior exploration is required before definitive stabilization.[2-5] Anterior dural tears also may occur, but they are not associated with nerve entrapment, and exploration is not necessary. If a tear is encountered during anterior decompression, however, it should be repaired primarily.[6] If this cannot be accomplished technically, a fibrin glue–type sealant can be used. Persistent leaks can be managed by subarachnoid drains. A drainage rate of 10 to 12 mL/h over 3 to 5 days usually is successful.[7]

Degree of Deformity

Some degree of deformity is common following thoracolumbar fractures, particularly with fractures associated with anterior compression or burst components. Although surgery can correct the deformity, in many instances the correction is at least partially lost over time, particularly with posterior surgery alone. Fortunately, there does not seem to be a correlation between deformity and functional outcome, especially for the stable burst fracture.[8,9] Because kyphotic deformities greater than 30° have been found to be associated with increased pain, these deformities should be considered for surgical correction and stabilization.[10]

Although some support exists in the literature for nonsurgical management of most burst fractures without neurologic deficit, the benefit of surgery in these patients is controversial.[11-13] Painful posttraumatic kyphosis may occur following injury and can be very difficult to treat.[14] These deformities commonly result from an unrecognized unstable injury, usually involving a component of distraction and/or rotational instability, or from failure of fixation. In a spinal cord injury, painful deformity also can result from the development of a Charcot spine.

Primary indications for surgery include progression of the deformity and/or a neurologic deficit as well as pain, although the success of surgery to primarily address pain is less predictable. Various authors have described surgical correction by an anterior-posterior procedure, an anterior procedure only, or a posterior osteotomy.[15-22] These procedures are effective, but they are also technically demanding, usually result in significant blood loss, and are associated with relatively high complication rates. With a Charcot spine, the patient may have neurologic changes such as decreased spasticity or a change in bladder function in addition to pain.[23] Arthrodesis has been used successfully to correct instability and deformity, restore sitting balance, and prevent complications resulting from neuropathic arthropathy.[24] In the presence of a Charcot spine, the approach usually involves combined anterior and posterior surgery.[25]

Gastrointestinal Problems

Various gastrointestinal problems may develop, and these are generally magnified in the presence of spinal cord injury. The incidence of ileus is increased with these injuries and becomes even more common after surgery and in the patient with a spinal cord injury. Close attention to bowel function and appropriate management of the diet are important. Stress-induced peptic ulcers can be associated with an increased trauma burden, especially when combined with early administration of a steroid infusion. Prophylactic use of histamine-2 (H2)-receptor blockers is recommended.

Simple constipation also is common and at times may be the patient's chief symptom. The combination of immobilization, spinal injury, possible concomitant abdominal injury, and the use of narcotics for pain control virtually guarantees problems with constipation. The judicious use of laxatives, appropriate diet, and early mobilization will help minimize this problem. Finally, in the presence of a spinal cord injury, a strict bowel management program is mandatory.[26] This is discussed further in chapter 12.

Neurologic mechanisms similar to those that control bowel function are responsible for bladder control.[26] In patients with a spinal cord injury, proper urodynamic evaluation is necessary to determine the best method of elimination, whether reflex mechanisms or self-catheterization. Again, a regular schedule is necessary to avoid complications of urinary tract infection and even autonomic dysreflexia. Urinary tract infections are a frequent source of significant morbidity in patients with spinal cord injuries.

Contractures and Decubitus Ulcers

Other complications associated with spinal cord injuries include contractures and decubitus ulcers, with the best approach for both being prevention. Spasticity and positioning can contribute to contractures, which significantly diminish a patient's functional potential. Management is discussed in chapter 12.

Decubitus ulcers can also substantially retard the rehabilitation process. Once present, they can be difficult to eradicate. Healing demands strict pressure relief, frequently including requiring the patient to avoid even such basic activities as sitting for extended periods of time. An appropriate mattress and frequent turning, especially in the acute and subacute stages of care, as well as vigilant inspection of the skin and early intervention will minimize skin breakdown. The rotating bed is still an effective means of preventing decubitus ulcers, particularly in patients with multiple traumatic injuries who may not be able to move for various reasons. A pressure relief brace may be useful, particularly in the distal lower extremities. Finally, if splinting or casting is required, especially in a limb with altered sensation or in a patient with altered mental status, the area must be very well padded and inspected frequently. To avoid external splinting, the early surgical stabilization of associated fractures is helpful.

Nutritional Deficiencies

Nutritional deficiencies can impede wound healing and the potential for rehabilitation. This is most often a problem in the patient with multiple traumatic injuries or a spinal cord injury. Serum albumin levels of less than 3.5 g/dL or total lymphocyte counts of less than 1,500 cells/mm^3 are standard assessments of nutritional deficiency. Depending on the condition of the patient, various interventions can be considered, from dietary nutritional supplements to enteral or total parenteral nutrition.

Deep Venous Thrombosis

The relation between thromboembolism and spinal injuries is poorly understood, and much current practice is not supported by the literature. Several authors have reviewed the incidence of deep venous thrombosis (DVT) and pulmonary embolus after spinal surgery.[27-33] These studies represent a very heterogeneous group of patients, ranging from those undergoing elective posterior surgery to anterior and posterior surgery to trauma patients and patients with a spinal cord injury. From these studies, several conclusions have been drawn. In general, the incidence of DVT and pulmonary embolus is higher in the presence of a spinal cord injury. The incidence of DVT in patients with a spinal cord injury varies from 49% to 100% in the first 12 weeks, with the highest rates occurring in the first 2 weeks. Maxwell and associates[33] found a significantly higher incidence in spinal cord injuries associated with concomitant long bone fractures. Anterior surgery is more likely to be associated with DVT. Finally, because some clots cause no symptoms, the incidence of DVT with spinal surgery is probably higher than initially thought, although the significance of these clinically silent clots is unknown.

Consensus is lacking regarding the use of prophylaxis for DVT in the postsurgical trauma patient without neurologic deficit. Although mechanical measures such as stockings and sequential compressive devices may not be sufficient, particularly when multiple risk factors such as age, anterior surgery, or multiple trauma are present, these measures are used liberally, admittedly without risk of additional harm. Hemorrhage is a possible side effect of chemical prophylaxis, and this is a particular concern following spinal surgery, especially acutely. If a clot is present in the acute postoperative period, placement of a vena cava filter should be seriously considered. A recent meta-analysis[34,35] reported that the risk of DVT was increased twofold with spinal trauma and threefold with spinal cord injury. The only other risk factor was increasing age. The pooled rates were 11.8% for DVT and 1.5% for pulmonary embolism. No method of DVT prophylaxis was found to be clearly superior to other methods or even to no prophylaxis.[35] However, when indicated, the use of a vena cava filter appeared to significantly reduce the incidence of pulmonary embolus. Particularly in the presence of a spinal cord injury, chemical prophylaxis is clearly recommended;[36] this is discussed further in chapter 12.

Pain

Chronic pain following thoracolumbar fractures, including osteoporotic fractures, is not uncommon and can result in significant disability.[37-39] Even in series reporting high functional recoveries, patients are often not pain free.[40] Patients who sustain these injuries should have realistic goals regarding recovery. The incidence of pain is higher in individuals with spinal cord injury, and neuropathic symptoms can be particularly recalcitrant and troublesome.[41,42] Management is discussed in chapter 12.

SURGICAL COMPLICATIONS

Posterior Surgical Treatment

Wrong-Site Surgery

One of the most elementary complications is wrong-site surgery. To avoid this, a thorough knowledge of spinal anatomy is necessary. Also, an appropriate marker radiograph should be obtained intraoperatively. Having a baseline radiograph available for comparison in the operating room, in addition to CT or MRI studies, is important to help minimize error in interpretation of these intraoperative radiographs. For the thoracolumbar area, the lateral marker radiograph should include the sacrum. If patient positioning and the operating room table permit, an AP view also may be obtained; preoperative comparison radiographs must be available because there can be anomalies in ribs or lumbar vertebrae. The relationships of these anomalies to the level of injury must be clearly understood, as simply identifying the site of the injury is not always clearly obvious.

Dural Tears

Dural tears were discussed more fully in the previous section. When an incidental durotomy occurs, the tear should be repaired primarily.[43] The addition of fibrin glue can also be considered.[44] If tears are addressed and repaired appropriately, no long-term sequelae are likely to occur.[45,46]

Neurologic Deficits

With any spinal surgery, it is important to examine the patient immediately upon awakening from anesthesia to assess for a change in neurologic status. This concern is heightened when the spine is unstable. Further neurologic damage can occur at various points, including during transfer to the operating room table, during positioning, and during the surgery, when direct trauma such as from inappropriate hardware placement, retraction of the spinal cord or conus, or rapid development of an epidural hematoma may occur.

In the patient with an unstable spine who has an incomplete injury or is intact neurologically, strong consideration should be given to spinal cord monitoring to provide continuous screening and to help prevent any iatrogenic causes of neurologic injury during surgery. This may be particularly helpful in patients with multiple traumatic injuries who remain intubated following surgery, making an examination impossible. If concerns arise in this circumstance, a wake-up test should be done if possible. Should the patient awaken with an increased deficit, the onus is on the surgeon to determine the cause immediately. If the deficit appears to be the result of spinal cord or conus medullaris injury, the evaluation must occur expeditiously. In some conditions, such as a spinal cord infarct, return to the operating room can be detrimental. Thus, if suspicions of a mechanical cause can be confirmed or dismissed quickly, these investigations should be completed rapidly. Depending on the hospital, in many cases, an imaging examination will not be possible before several hours have passed, so strong consideration should be given to immediate return to the operating room for careful exploration and assessment, including hardware removal and evaluation of decompression. During this procedure, arrangements can be made to obtain immediate postoperative imaging.

When neurologic deficit is present, MRI is the initial study of choice, even in the presence of hardware; most instrumentation is made of titanium, so the artifact usually is not severe enough to interfere with a good interpretation of the neurologic structures. CT provides more bone detail than MRI and is a more accurate measure of hardware placement. Myelography can provide indirect information regarding excessive neural compression. If a nerve root deficit is suspected, the situation is less urgent. The workup should proceed expeditiously, but unless intraoperative radiographs indicate a clear need for revision, a definitive diagnosis should be obtained before returning to the operating room.

Blood Loss

Control of blood loss can be difficult with spinal surgery, and even more so in the presence of acute trauma. Positioning is important, and good decompression of the abdomen will help control bleeding to a degree. An additional strategy often used by the surgeon is to maintain a reduced intraoperative blood pressure. This is contraindicated, however, in the presence of a neurologic deficit, in which case systolic blood pressures should be maintained above 85 to 90 mm Hg. Even if the spinal cord is intact, consideration should be given to minimizing reduction of blood pressure intraoperatively if the spine is unstable. The use of a cell saver has been shown to be efficacious during surgery for acute spinal trauma in helping with blood salvage.[47]

Iliac Crest Bone Graft

For posterior surgery, a posterior iliac crest bone graft is still the gold standard. Various types of complications have been reported, but this is a generally safe procedure. Most complications are minor, with the most common being postoperative pain.[48,49] Although the pain usually dissipates with time, patients should be advised that this is a possibility with this procedure. Posterior graft pain tends to be less severe and less common than anterior graft pain. Additionally, the incidence of significant pain seems to be considerably higher after elective reconstruction than after trauma surgery.[50] Deep infections are rare and are usually managed successfully with prompt and aggressive irrigation and débridement. Injury to cluneal nerves can be avoided by staying within 6 cm of the posterior superior iliac spine.[51] This can be easily accomplished by making a more vertically directed incision centered near the posterior superior iliac spine versus an oblique incision. Severe complications such as pelvic fracture, sciatic nerve injury, and superior gluteal artery injury are exceedingly rare. If a laceration to the artery occurs, access can be obtained by extending the posterior exposure, thus avoiding having to turn the patient.[52]

Unrecognized Injuries

Understanding the mechanism of injury is important because failure to recognize certain injuries, particularly distraction or rotational injuries, may result in delayed neurologic deficits.[53] Fractures that require surgical stabilization usually also require some type of reduction. The first feature to look for is the presence of a posterior distraction mechanism. These injuries should not be distracted to obtain a concomitant anterior fracture reduction because this could result in undesirable neurologic injury. In the case of a burst fracture that is the result of a flexion-distraction injury, the corrective force should emphasize lordosis without distraction. In the case of a compression burst injury, lordosis and distraction can be used for indirect reduction. In a laminar fracture, absence of a dural tear with nerve root entrapment should be established before reduction.

Inadequate Decompression

There is some debate regarding the desired degree of decompression, particularly in the presence of a neurologic deficit. In this situation, goals usually include a thorough decompression of the spinal canal. Direct decompression anteriorly has been shown to be more complete and reliable than indirect posterior reduction.[54] However, the benefit of an extensive decompression is controversial. Some studies show that neurologic recovery has no correlation with the magnitude of spinal canal compromise,[55-59] but other reports indicate that neurologic improvement does follow additional decompression.[60-63] Thus, the degree to which failure of reduction to achieve decompression should be regarded as a complication is uncertain. It would certainly appear to be less important in the neurologically intact patient.

Instrumentation Failure

With the progressive development of implant systems, the use of instrumentation has increased, thereby increasing the risk of hardware-related complications. The use of pedicle screws has been associated with a variety of problems.[64] Initial reports showed a higher rate of screw-related neurologic problems,[65,66] but recent studies suggest that few problems are associated with placement of the screws when they are inserted under the guidance of experienced surgeons.[67,68] The use of electrical stimulation devices to check proximity of hardware to nerves can help improve clinical safety.[69,70] Postoperative symptoms are usually best evaluated with CT myelography. The process of placing pedicle screws can cause a dural tear. Most tears do not require repair, especially if there is no plan for open posterior decompression. Using the same screw entry site if possible, the instrumentation can be appropriately redirected or the hole can be plugged with bone graft or bone wax. Anecdotally, this seems to be effective and have no sequelae. If there is a visible leak of cerebrospinal fluid from an adjacent decompressed area, the tear should be explored and repaired.

Frequently, some loss of correction of alignment occurs with posterior instrumentation alone. Hardware failure also has been reported, although this is not necessarily associated with poor outcomes.[71,72] When loss of correction is of concern, the posterior short pedicle screw constructs can be strengthened by additional sublaminar hooks[73] or by additional levels of fixation,[74] or consideration can be given to anterior constructs.[75]

Pneumothorax may arise following posterior procedures as the result of aberrant instrumentation procedures or traumatic pleural disruption, particularly in the case of a rotationally unstable injury. Postoperative radiographs of the chest should be obtained following placement of thoracic pedicle screws, particularly if any difficulty was encountered during placement that would heighten suspicion for a pleural injury.

Pseudarthrosis

Although pseudarthrosis can occur following attempted arthrodesis, the incidence appears to be much less than that observed with elective fusions. From their own work, as well as a review of the literature, Edwards and Levine[76] reported an incidence of pseudarthrosis of about 4% in a trauma population. Known contributory factors include anti-inflammatory drugs, smoking, advanced age, and poor nutrition.[77-79] Accurate assessment of fusion is difficult without surgical exploration. Evaluation tools primarily consist of AP, lateral, and flexion-extension radiographs and/or CT. Even after extensive imaging and especially in the presence of hardware, uncertainty may persist regarding the status of the fusion. Careful judgment must be exercised in the patient with persistent pain. It is easy to assume that the pseudarthrosis is responsible for pain, but nonunion does not necessarily affect outcomes.[80] A thorough investigation of all possible sources of pain must be conducted, along with a prolonged course of nonsurgical rehabilitation, before considering any surgical revision for pain. The primary concerns related to a pseudarthrosis are progression of deformity and/or neurologic deficit. These are considered indications for revision surgery, and management of progressive deformity is discussed above. For prevention of nonunion at the index procedure, autogenous bone graft and the use of instrumentation appear to be effective.[81]

Infection

The trauma patient seems to be at increased risk for postoperative infection. The authors of a recent study comparing the rate of postoperative spinal infections in trauma patients with that in patients undergoing elective surgery over a 3-year period[82] reported that the infection rate in the trauma patients was nearly three times that of the elective patients (9.4% versus 3.7%). Surgical delays and longer stays in the intensive care unit postoperatively were found to be significant risk factors. Other factors, such as associated acute comorbidities and nutrition, may also play a role. Once again, prevention is the best treatment. Administration of perioperative antibiotics is mandatory. The first dose should be given within 1 hour of the incision and repeated at half the otherwise usual dosing interval. All trauma patients should be scrubbed with an antiseptic soap for several minutes before the formal surgical preparation.

Early recognition of infection is of critical importance. A promptly treated deep infection is very curable, but delayed intervention can result in conditions that may be difficult to correct. When an acute infection presents late with an established fusion, hardware removal is recommended, along with irrigation, débridement, and antibiotics. When infection occurs during the earlier postoperative period, when the fusion mass has not yet matured, the hardware can be retained as long as the infection is addressed promptly with surgery. Irrigation and débridement must be performed, sometimes on multiple occasions. Other strategies include primary closure over a drain or with antibiotic beads, primary closure over a continuous antibiotic irrigation and suction system, or delayed closure with or without a flap.[83-86] Long-term, culture-specific antibiotics are also administered. The antibiotic course is somewhat dependent on intraoperative findings, history of the infection, and type of organism. The most common organism continues to be *Staphylococcus*. If these principles are adhered to, chances are good for eradication of infection and progression to solid arthrodesis.

Anterior Surgical Treatment

Anterior and posterior procedures share several complications, including dural tears, neurologic deficits, hardware failure, pseudarthrosis, loss of correction or progression of deformity, and infection, and they are managed similarly, regardless of the approach. However, several complications are unique to the anterior approach.

Complications Associated With Thoracotomy

Thoracolumbar fractures nearly always require a thoracotomy, usually with incision of the diaphragm. In general, postthoracotomy pain seems to be better tolerated than the pain associated with the posterior approach to the spine, although initial rehabilitation can be more protracted because a chest tube is present and more difficulties associated with pulmonary function develop. Injury can occur to an intercostal nerve, resulting in a paresthesia that is annoying to the patient but rarely of functional consequence. Because of the mechanisms of injury common with thoracolumbar fractures, associated chest injuries such as pneumothorax, pulmonary contusions, and rib fractures commonly occur. In the presence of these comorbidities, a thoracotomy may be contraindicated, depending on the underlying health status of the patient. Performing a thoracotomy in these circumstances could place the patient at unreasonable risk for further pulmonary compromise. In this situation, an initial posterior procedure can be considered to allow for initial stabilization and mobilization. Further anterior stability may be accomplished after the patient recovers from the initial pulmonary injuries.

Visceral Injuries

Various visceral injuries can occur. In thoracolumbar fractures, injury to the ureter occurs rarely because of the level of exposure, but if there is a laceration, it should be repaired directly. A breach of the peritoneum can occur during exposure; this should be repaired primarily. If the tear is large, failure to repair it adequately can result in herniation of the bowel and resultant obstruction. Also rare are thoracic duct injuries, which may be iatrogenic or the result of the force of the initial injury.[87] These are usually recognized on a delayed basis, especially once the patient starts to eat, when milky drainage is observed. The presence of this drainage may be confused with infection initially. Initial management usually consists of observation. Occasionally, a persistent leak will require exploration and repair.

Vascular Injuries

Several vessels are at risk for injury. Tears of the azygos or hemiazygos vein can be ligated. Lacerations of the vena cava or aorta must be repaired. Concerns have been raised regarding sacrificing segmental vessels in the lower thoracic area. In theory, interruption of a dominant vessel can result in ischemic injury to the spinal cord. However, in 1,197 patients who underwent anterior deformity surgery,[88] no incidences of paraplegia were found, although this was for elective deformity. If there is concern, the vessels can be occluded temporarily before ligation with concurrent spinal cord monitoring. If loss of signal is detected, ligation of the segmental vessels can then be avoided.

SUMMARY AND CONCLUSIONS

Clearly, management of thoracolumbar fractures can be very difficult. Numerous complications can arise not only secondary to surgery but also from the actual injury itself. Many of these complications can be minimized if not prevented by anticipating their occurrence. Several other complications are very manageable, and early recognition usually facilitates effective treatment. A thorough awareness and expectation of these various complications results in optimal postinjury care.

REFERENCES

1. Knop C, Bastian L, Lange U, Oeser M, Zdichavsky M, Blauth M: Complications in surgical treatment of thoracolumbar injuries. *Eur Spine J* 2002; 11:214-226.
2. Aydinli U, Karaeminogullari O, Tiskaya K, Ozturk C: Dural tears in lumbar burst fractures with greenstick lamina fractures. *Spine* 2001;26:E410-E415.
3. Cammisa FP, Eismont FJ, Green BA: Dural laceration occurring with burst fractures and associated laminar fractures. *J Bone Joint Surg Am* 1989;71:1044-1052.
4. Denis F, Burkus JK: Diagnosis and treatment of cauda equina entrapment in the vertical lamina fracture of lumbar burst fractures. *Spine* 1991;16:S433-S439.
5. Keenen TL, Antony J, Benson DR: Dural tears associated with lumbar burst fractures. *J Orthop Trauma* 1990;4:243-245.
6. Carl AL, Matsumoto M, Whalen JT: Anterior dural laceration caused by thoracolumbar and lumbar burst fractures. *J Spinal Disord* 2000;13:399-403.
7. Kitchel SH, Eismont FJ, Green BA: Closed subarachnoid drainage for management of cerebrospinal fluid leakage after an operation on the spine. *J Bone Joint Surg Am* 1989;71:984-987.
8. Cantor JB, Lebwohl NH, Garvey T, Eismont FJ: Nonoperative management of stable thoracolumbar burst fractures with early ambulation and bracing. *Spine* 1993;18:971-976.
9. Mumford J, Weinstein JN, Spratt KF, Goel VK: Thoracolumbar burst fractures: The clinical efficacy and outcome of nonoperative management. *Spine* 1993;18:955-970.
10. Gertzbein SD: Scoliosis Research Society: Multicenter spine fracture study. *Spine* 1992;17:528-540.
11. Denis F, Armstrong GW, Searls K, Matta L: Acute thoracolumbar burst fractures in the absence of neurologic deficit: A comparison between operative and nonoperative treatment. *Clin Orthop* 1984;189:142-149.

12. Shen WJ, Liu TJ, Shen YS: Nonoperative treatment versus posterior fixation for thoracolumbar junction burst fractures without neurologic deficit. *Spine* 2001;26:1038-1045.

13. Wood K, Butterman G, Mehbod A, Garvery T, Jhanjee R, Sechriest V: Operative compared with nonoperative treatment of a thoracolumbar burst fracture without neurological deficit: A prospective, randomized study. *J Bone Joint Surg Am* 2003;85:773-781.

14. Vaccaro AR, Silber JS: Post-traumatic spinal deformity. *Spine* 2001;26(suppl):S111-S118.

15. Bridwell KH, Lenke LG, Lewis SJ: Treatment of spinal stenosis and fixed sagittal imbalance. *Clin Orthop* 2001;384:35-44.

16. Gertzbein SD, Harris MB: Wedge osteotomy for the correction of post-traumatic kyphosis. *Spine* 1992;17:374-379.

17. Gertzbein SD, Hollopeter MR, Hall S: Pseudarthrosis of the lumbar spine: Outcome after circumferential fusion. *Spine* 1998;23:2352-2357.

18. Kostuik JP, Maurais GR, Richardson WJ, Okajima Y: Combined single stage anterior and posterior osteotomy for correction of iatrogenic lumbar kyphosis. *Spine* 1988;13:257-266.

19. Kostuik JP, Matsusaki H: Anterior stabilization, instrumentation, and decompression for post-traumatic kyphosis. *Spine* 1989;14:379-386.

20. Murrey DB, Brigham CD, Kiebzak GM, Finger F, Chewning SJ: Transpedicular decompression and pedicle subtraction osteotomy (eggshell procedure): A retrospective review of 59 patients. *Spine* 2002;27:2338-2345.

21. Malcolm BW, Bradford DS, Winter RB, Chou SN: Post-traumatic kyphosis: A review of forty-eight surgically treated patients. *J Bone Joint Surg Am* 1981;63:891-899.

22. Wu SS: Hwa Sy, Lin LC, Pai WM, Chen PQ, Au MK: Management of rigid post-traumatic kyphosis. *Spine* 1996;21:2260-2267.

23. Standaert C, Cardenas DD, Anderson P: Charcot spine as a late complication of traumatic spinal cord injury. *Arch Phys Med Rehabil* 1997;78:221-225.

24. Sobel JW, Bohlman HH, Freehafer AA: Charcot's arthropathy of the spine following spinal cord injury: A report of five cases. *J Bone Joint Surg Am* 1985;67:771-776.

25. Brown CW, Jones B, Donaldson DH, Akmakjian J, Brugman JL: Neuropathic (Charcot) arthropathy of the spine after traumatic spinal paraplegia. *Spine* 1992;17(suppl):S103-S108.

26. Apple DF: Medical management and rehabilitation of the spinal cord injured patient, in Cotler JM, Simpson JM, An HS, Silveri CP (eds): *Surgery of Spinal Trauma*. Philadelphia, PA, Lippincott Williams & Wilkins, 2000, pp 157-178.

27. Dearborn JT, Hu SS, Tribus CB, Bradford DS: Thromboembolic complications after major thoracolumbar spine surgery. *Spine* 1999;24:1471-1476.

28. Oda T, Fuji T, Kato Y, Fujita S, Kanemitsu N: Deep venous thrombosis after posterior spinal surgery. *Spine* 2000;25:2962-2967.

29. Rokito SE, Schwartz MC, Neuwirth MG: Deep vein thrombosis after major reconstructive spinal surgery. *Spine* 1996;21:853-859.

30. Smith MD, Bressler EL, Lonstein JE, Winter R, Pinto MR, Denis F: Deep venous thrombosis and pulmonary embolism after major reconstructive operations on the spine: A prospective analysis of three hundred and seventeen patients. *J Bone Joint Surg Am* 1994;76:980-985.

31. West JL III, Anderson LD: Incidence of deep vein thrombosis in major adult spinal surgery. *Spine* 1992;17(suppl):S254-S257.

32. Merli GJ, Crabbe S, Paluzzi RG, Fritz D: Etiology, incidence, and prevention of deep vein thrombosis in acute spinal cord injury. *Arch Phys Med Rehabil* 1993;74:1199-1205.

33. Maxwell RA, Chavarria-Aguilar M, Cockerham WT, et al: Routine prophylactic vena cava filtration is not indicated after acute spinal cord injury. *J Trauma* 2002;52:902-906.

34. Velmahos GC, Kern J, Chan LS, Oder D, Murray JA, Shekelle P: Prevention of venous thromboembolism after injury: An evidence-based report. Part II: Analysis of risk factors and evaluation of the role of vena caval filters. *J Trauma* 2000;49:140-144.

35. Velmahos GC, Kern J, Chan LS, Oder D, Murray JA, Shekelle P: Prevention of venous thromboembolism after injury: An evidence-based report. Part I: Analysis of risk factors and evaluation of the role of vena caval filters. *J Trauma* 2000;49:132-139.

36. Green D, Hull RD, Mammen EF, Merli GJ, Weingarden SI, Yao JS: Deep vein thrombosis in spinal cord injury: Summary and recommendations. *Chest* 1992;102(suppl):633S-635S.

37. Kraemer WJ, Schemitsch EH, Lever J, McBroom RJ, McKee MD, Waddell JP: Functional outcome of thoracolumbar burst fractures without neurological deficit. *J Orthop Trauma* 1996;10:541-544.

38. Tasdemiroglu E, Tibbs PA: Long-term follow-up results of thoracolumbar fractures after posterior instrumentation. *Spine* 1995;20:1704-1708.

39. Nguyen HV, Ludwig S, Gelb D: Osteoporotic vertebral burst fractures with neurologic compromise. *J Spinal Disord Tech* 2003;16:10-19.

40. Weinstein JN, Collalto P, Lehmann TR: Thoracolumbar "burst" fractures treated conservatively: A long-term follow-up. *Spine* 1988;13:33-38.

41. Fenollosa P, Pallares J, Cervera J, et al: Chronic pain in the spinal cord injured: Statistical approach and pharmacological treatment. *Paraplegia* 1993;31:722-729.

42. Ravenscroft A, Ahmed YS, Burnside IG: Chronic pain after SCI: A patient survey. *Spinal Cord* 2000;38:611-614.

43. Eismont FJ, Wiesel SW, Rothman RH: Treatment of dural tears associated with spinal surgery. *J Bone Joint Surg Am* 1981;63:1132-1136.

44. Cain JE, Dryer RF, Barton BR: Evaluation of dural closure techniques: Suture methods, fibrin adhesive sealant, and cyanoacrylate polymer. *Spine* 1988;13:720-725.

45. Cammisa FP, Girardi FP, Sangani PK, Parvataneni HK, Cadag S, Sandhu HS: Incidental durotomy in spine surgery. *Spine* 2000;25:2663-2667.

46. Wang JC, Bohlman HH, Riew KD: Dural tears secondary to operations on the lumbar spine: Management and results after a two-year minimum follow-up of eighty-eight patients. *J Bone Joint Surg Am* 1998;80:1728-1732.

47. Cavallieri S, Riou B, Roche S, Ducart A, Roy-Camille R, Viars P: Intraoperative autologous transfusion in emergency surgery for spine trauma. *J Trauma* 1994;36:639-643.

48. Banwart JC, Asher MA, Hassanein RS: Iliac crest bone graft harvest donor site morbidity: A statistical evaluation. *Spine* 1995;20:1055-1060.

49. Robertson PA, Wray AC: Natural history of posterior iliac crest bone graft donation for spinal surgery: A prospective analysis of morbidity. *Spine* 2001;26:1473-1476.

50. Fernyhough JC, Schimandle JJ, Weigel MC, et al: Chronic donor site pain complicating bone graft harvesting from the posterior iliac crest for spinal fusion. *Spine* 1992;17:1474-1480.

51. Xu R, Ebraheim NA, Yeasting RA, Jackson WT: Anatomic considerations for posterior iliac bone harvesting. *Spine* 1996;21:1017-1020.

52. Shin AY, Moran ME, Wenger DR: Superior gluteal artery injury secondary to posterior iliac crest bone graft harvesting: A surgical technique to control hemorrhage. *Spine* 1996;21:1371-1374.

53. Gertzbein SD: Neurologic deterioration in patients with thoracic and lumbar fractures after admission to the hospital. *Spine* 1994;19:1723-1725.

54. Esses SI, Botsford DJ, Wright T, Bednar D, Bailey S: Operative treatment of spinal fractures with the AO internal fixator. *Spine* 1991;16(suppl):S146-S150.

55. Boerger TO, Limb D, Dickson RA: Does "canal clearance" affect neurological outcome after thoracolumbar burst fractures? *J Bone Joint Surg Br* 2000;82:629-635.

56. Crutcher JP, Anderson PA, King HA, Montesano PX: Indirect spinal canal decompression in patients with thoracolumbar burst fractures treated by posterior distraction rods. *J Spinal Disord* 1991;4:39-48.

57. Herndon WA, Galloway D: Neurologic return versus cross-sectional canal area in incomplete thoracolumbar spinal cord injuries. *J Trauma* 1988;28:680-683.

58. Mohanty SP, Venkatram N: Does neurological recovery in thoracolumbar and lumbar burst fractures depend on the extent of canal compromise? *Spinal Cord* 2002;40:295-299.

59. Shuman WP, Rogers JV, Sickler ME, et al: Thoracolumbar burst fractures: CT dimensions of the spinal canal relative to postsurgical improvement. *AJR Am J Roentgenol* 1985;145:337-341.

60. Bohlman HH, Kirkpatrick JS, Delamarter RB, Leventhal M: Anterior decompression for late pain and paralysis after fractures of the thoracolumbar spine. *Clin Orthop* 1994;300:24-29.

61. Bradford DS, McBride GG: Surgical management of thoracolumbar spine fractures with incomplete neurologic deficits. *Clin Orthop* 1987;218:201-216.

62. McAfee PC, Bohlman HH, Yuan HA: Anterior decompression of traumatic thoracolumbar fractures with incomplete neurological deficit using a retroperitoneal approach. *J Bone Joint Surg Am* 1985;67:89-104.

63. Transfeldt EE, White D, Bradford DS, Roche B: Delayed anterior decompression in patients with spinal cord and cauda equina injuries of the thoracolumbar spine. *Spine* 1990;15:953-957.

64. Esses SI, Sachs B, Dreyzin V: Complications associated with the technique of pedicle screw fixation: A selected survey of ABS members. *Spine* 1993;18:2231-2239.

65. Castro WH, Halm H, Jerosch J, Malms J, Steinbeck J, Blasius S: Accuracy of pedicle screw placement in lumbar vertebrae. *Spine* 1996;21:1320-1324.

66. Yuan HA, Garfin SR, Dickman CA, Mardjetko SM: A historical cohort study of pedicle screw fixation in thoracic, lumbar, and sacral spinal fusions. *Spine* 1994;19(suppl):2279S-2296S.

67. Belmont PT, Klemme WR, Robinson M, Polly DW: Accuracy of thoracic pedicle screws in patients with and without coronal plane spinal deformities. *Spine* 2002;27:1558-1566.

68. Lonstein JE, Denis F, Perra JH, Pinto MR, Smith MD, Winter RB: Complications associated with pedicle screws. *J Bone Joint Surg Am* 1999;81:1519-1528.

69. Glassman SD, Dimar JR, Puno RM, Johnson JR, Shields CB, Linden RD: A prospective analysis of intraoperative electromyographic monitoring of pedicle screw placement with computed tomographic scan confirmation. *Spine* 1995;20:1375-1379.

70. Shi YB, Binette M, Martin WH, Pearson JM, Hart RA: Electrical stimulation for intraoperative evaluation of thoracic pedicle screw placement. *Spine* 2003;28:595-601.

71. Gaebler C, Maier R, Kukla C, Vecsei V: Long-term results of pedicle stabilized thoracolumbar fractures in relation to the neurological deficit. *Injury* 1997;28:661-666.

72. McLain RF, Sparling E, Benson DR: Early failure of short-segment pedicle instrumentation for thoracolumbar fractures: A preliminary report. *J Bone Joint Surg Am* 1993;75:162-167.

73. Chiba M, McLain RF, Yerby SA, Moseley TA, Smith TS, Benson DR: Short-segment pedicle instrumentation: Biomechanical analysis of supplemental hook fixation. *Spine* 1996;21:288-294.

74. Katonis PG, Kontakis GM, Loupasis GA, Aligizakis AC, Christoforakis JI, Velivassakis EG: Treatment of unstable thoracolumbar and lumbar spine injuries using Cotrel-Dubousset instrumentation. *Spine* 1999;24:2352-2357.

75. Parker JW, Lane JR, Karaikovic EE, Gaines RW: Successful short-segment instrumentation and fusion for thoracolumbar spine fractures: A consecutive 4 1/2-year series. *Spine* 2000;25:1157-1170.

76. Edwards CC, Levine AM: Complications associated with posterior instrumentation in the treatment of thoracic and lumbar injuries, in Garfin S (ed): *Complications of Spine Surgery*. Baltimore, MD, Williams & Wilkins, 1989, pp 164-199.

77. Klein JD, Hey LA, Yu CS, et al: Perioperative nutrition and postoperative complications in patients undergoing spinal surgery. *Spine* 1996;21:2676-2682.

78. Glassman SD, Anagnost SC, Parker A, Burke D, Johnson JR, Dimar JR: The effect of cigarette smoking and smoking cessation on spinal fusion. *Spine* 2000;25:2608-2615.

79. Glassman SD, Rose SM, Dimar JR, Puno RM, Campbell MJ, Johnson JR: The effect of postoperative nonsteroidal anti-inflammatory drug administration on spinal fusion. *Spine* 1998;23:834-838.

80. Fischgrund JS, Mackay M, Herkowitz HN, Brower R, Montgomery DM, Kurz LT: Degenerative lumbar spondylolisthesis with spinal stenosis: A prospective, randomized study comparing decompressive laminectomy and arthrodesis with and without spinal instrumentation. *Spine* 1997;22:2807-2812.

81. Zdeblick TA: A prospective, randomized study of lumbar fusion: Preliminary results. *Spine* 1993;18:983-991.

82. Blam OG, Vaccaro AR, Vanichkachorn JS, et al: Risk factors for surgical site infection in the patient with spinal injury. *Spine* 2003;28:1475-1480.

83. Dumanian GA, Ondra SL, Liu J, Schafer MF, Chao JD: Muscle flap salvage of spine wounds with soft tissue defects or infection. *Spine* 2003;28:1203-1211.

84. Levi AD, Dickman CA, Sonntag VK: Management of postoperative infections after spinal instrumentation. *J Neurosurg* 1997;86:975-980.

85. Stambough JL, Beringer D: Postoperative wound infections complicating adult spine surgery. *J Spinal Disord* 1992;5:277-285.

86. Weinstein MA, McCabe JP, Cammisa FP: Postoperative spinal wound infection: A review of 2,391 consecutive index procedures. *J Spinal Disord* 2000;13:422-426.

87. Silen ML, Weber TR: Management of thoracic duct injury associated with fracture-dislocation of the spine following blunt trauma. *J Trauma* 1995;39:1185-1187.

88. Winter RB, Lonstein JE, Denis F, Leonard AS, Garamella JJ: Paraplegia resulting from vessel ligation. *Spine* 1996;21:1232-1234.

CHAPTER 14

SUMMARY AND CONCLUSIONS

CHARLES A. REITMAN, MD

The management of thoracolumbar fractures continues to evolve. In general, outcomes have improved as a result of advances in the response to trauma, with care now being more expeditious, more thorough, and more complete. At the newer high-level trauma centers, life-threatening injuries are recognized and managed more quickly, and initial stabilization of patients with multiple injuries is optimized. As a result, patients with very complex injuries are recovering and returning to productive lives.

This monograph presents a comprehensive review of the management of thoracolumbar fractures. Strong consensus exists regarding some aspects of care, but in other areas, significant controversy remains. This chapter presents my bias in treating these injuries.

INITIAL EVALUATION

Maintaining a high index of suspicion in all patients is of utmost importance for both the trauma surgeon and the spine surgeon. Most spinal injuries result from blunt trauma, which frequently causes multiple distracting injuries that can mask a spinal fracture.[1] Every patient who has sustained a significant fall or collision must undergo a thorough physical examination after initial evaluation and stabilization. Every bone must be palpated, every limb moved. A detailed and complete neurologic examination must be conducted, including assessment of strength, sensation, deep tendon reflexes, long tract signs, and rectal sphincter tone. Despite the availability of increasingly sophisticated imaging modalities, some of the most useful information for surgical decision making and predicting outcomes still comes from the preinjury baseline condition of the patient and the physical examination. If the patient cannot cooperate, the assessment should be completed to the extent possible, and it is mandatory that the patient undergo a complete examination when they can cooperate, whether 1 hour or 1 month later. Missed injuries are common, especially in patients who are obtunded. I believe that the outcome of many musculoskeletal injuries can be improved by intervention even weeks or months after onset. Thus, ongoing evaluation is necessary until the patient's condition is completely understood.

Imaging

With any suspicion of a spinal injury, AP and lateral radiographs of the relevant area of the vertebral column should be obtained. If a spinal fracture is discovered, radiographs of the entire vertebral column should be obtained because noncontiguous fractures are not uncommon.[2] In the obtunded patient with a significant mechanism of injury, AP and lateral views of the entire spine should be obtained. In the areas of suspicion, CT should be used to image all levels not visualized on radiographs as well as all areas in which a fracture is apparent on radiographs.[3-5]

The trend at some institutions is to use CT for all initial imaging.[6] The new spiral CT scanners are extremely fast, and it is often more efficient to perform a total body CT scan early in the evaluation process. I believe that plain radiographs are still useful in decision making and certainly in long-term follow-up. However, the total body CT scan provides good detail regarding alignment, and in combination with thin-cut axial CT scans and CT reconstructions, it provides extremely useful and accurate information in a very expeditious manner, facilitating care of the patient in several ways. It allows the orthopaedic surgeon and the trauma team to make decisions and dispositions quickly, to get the patient off the backboard in a timely manner, to allow continued care by other services with appropriate precautions, and to expedite the overall emergency workup. In addition to expediting care, most importantly it will likely improve the quality of care. The use of CT should not result in increased missed injuries, and in fact there are some early data to support the idea that CT will reduce the number of missed injuries. The more severe the overall trauma, the more justified and efficient the total body CT scan is. This is because the likelihood that an injury will be diagnosed with CT increases with the severity of the mechanism of injury. This is true for the spine as well as other systems. Concerns about radiation exposure and cost must be addressed.[7,8]

Steroid Treatment

At my institution, we use the methylprednisolone continuous infusion as outlined in the third National Acute Spinal Cord Injury Study (NASCIS III).[9] I am strict about not using steroids if they have not been started within 8 hours of the injury, but this is rarely overlooked. I always administer a gastroprotectant. I believe that in the near future, other pharmacologic strategies will probably replace steroids or be combined with them,[10] as research in this area is very active. In general, I do not administer steroids to patients with penetrating trauma.

CONSIDERATIONS WITH TRANSVERSE PROCESS FRACTURES

The most common fractures seen at my institution are transverse process fractures. These fractures are generally benign, but they are a sign of a significant mechanism of injury and are frequently associated with abdominal or pelvic injuries. Because it is tempting to be complacent when presented with a transverse process fracture, the surgeon must have a high index of suspicion for associated injuries, particularly contiguous spinous process and transverse process fractures. This fracture combination may be a subtle indication of a rotational mechanism, so when it is present, further investigation is indicated to rule out an unstable rotational injury.

STABLE VERSUS UNSTABLE INJURIES

One of the longest chapters in this monograph is on biomechanics, reflecting the fact that debate continues as to what constitutes a stable injury. Part of the difficulty is the use of static imaging to assess a dynamic problem. This uncertainty is especially problematic given that the surgeon's understanding of spinal instability usually determines the choice between surgical and nonsurgical treatment.

General guidelines exist for what constitutes a stable injury. For example, ligamentous injuries are generally thought to be unstable and prone to progressive deformity and pain. However, it is not uncommon to see patients with missed injuries or with injuries that caused spinal surgery to be delayed for weeks or months who are successfully treated nonsurgically. As another example, it is suggested that burst injuries with more than 50% canal compromise or 50% collapse of vertebral height are unstable. However, depending particularly on the level of injury, again it is not uncommon to see patients with injuries exceeding these parameters who are treated successfully without surgery. Conversely, I have seen progressive deformity in patients who presented on a delayed basis with no apparent ligamentous injury and an "acceptable" initial deformity.

Given these uncertainties, the question of who needs to be stabilized is not easy to answer. I agree with other authors in this monograph that patients who have a neurologic deficit with a spinal fracture due to blunt trauma probably warrant surgery. Regardless of the existing deformity or canal stenosis, substantial deformity must have been present initially to cause a neurologic deficit.[11] Some evidence exists that patients with incomplete deficits who are treated surgically recover better function long term.[12-14] There is no question that it is easier to manage multiple injuries once the patient has been stabilized. Surgery in this case would include both a decompression and fusion. In the presence of a progressive neurologic deficit, surgery must proceed as immediately as possible, depending on the status of other more life-threatening injuries. If the neurologic examination is stable, no convincing evidence exists in humans that proceeding with immediate decompression makes a difference in the outcome, although animal studies suggest that early decompression is beneficial.[15-17] Early stabilization does allow for earlier mobilization and therefore potentially faster rehabilitation and fewer complications related to bed rest. I do not believe that these patients require emergent surgery, but I still prefer to perform surgery as soon as possible, depending on the availability of the operating room and appropriate staff, usually within the first 24 hours postinjury as long as other medical issues allow. Patients with severe multiple injuries also are likely to benefit from early intervention.[18]

Surgical Approach

Once the decision has been made to operate, a decision has to be made as to anterior approach, posterior approach, or both. In a patient with a neurologic deficit, decompression can certainly be accomplished with either approach, and as long as the goals of surgery are attained, the choice often becomes one of personal preference. If the injury is a compression-only mechanism (type A fracture in the comprehensive classification system described in chapter 3), I generally decompress and stabilize anteriorly only. Some studies have shown that the decompression is better and the neurologic recovery is possibly better with an interior approach than with indirect posterior decompression.[19-21] The fusion is a compression graft, which is very stable and typically has a low incidence of long-term progressive deformity.[21] I prefer to use a nonexpendable mesh vertical cage and a staple device with dual rods. I use autograft from the vertebral body as well as the rib if it is harvested, which is virtually always adequate. Many other reasonable options exist for the strut graft as well as the implant.

If a distraction or rotational component is present, the strategy is completely different, which is why it is so important not to miss a distraction injury. Distraction injuries (type B injuries in the comprehensive classification) need to be stabilized with a posterior approach because of the disruption of the tension band. Reduction of a dislocation also requires a posterior approach. Decompression can be accomplished with laminectomy and a footed tamp on the posteriorly displaced fragments that do not reduce with ligamentotaxis. Caution is required in the region of the conus or spinal cord. I essentially always use pedicle screw fixation because I believe this provides the best control and fixation. It also usually allows the minimum levels of fixation, especially inferiorly, where it is an advantage to minimize the number of lumbar levels fused. Occasional exceptions include anatomic variations or the presence of highly osteoporotic bone. A critical review of the preoperative CT scan will help the surgeon judge pedicle size and decide how the implants will be placed.

Loss of correction is a concern with posterior-only surgery.[22] To maintain short segment fixation, an alternative fixation strategy is to use pedicle screws and inferior laminar hooks at the lumbar level below and pedicle screws at two levels above.[23] This provides slightly better mechanical advantage without additional loss of important lumbar motion segments. The main initial goal, however, is stabilization and fusion. Thus, if there is any concern regarding adequacy of fixation, a level should be added to the construct.

If the intraoperative results are satisfactory, as determined both by what is observed in the wound and by radiographs, the surgery can be limited to the posterior procedure. In the case of a distraction injury with a burst component, however, I recommend a postoperative CT scan to determine if substantial stenosis remains, in which case a supplemental anterior procedure is warranted. If no anterior structural support remains because of the impaction of the compression, as in the higher grade fractures described by McCormack,[24] a supplemental anterior procedure also can be considered, particularly if there is a short segment fusion posteriorly.[25] For posterior followed by anterior fusion, my choice for the anterior strut is either an allograft strut or a mesh cage with local autograft. The second procedure can be delayed for several days if necessary. The patient can mobilize with the posterior procedure alone, and delaying the anterior procedure can even make things easier in terms of intraoperative blood loss and visibility. However, if I am certain at the outset that I will proceed with an anterior procedure as well, I prefer to do both at the same time if the posterior procedure goes well. The only reason to do a staged procedure, other than a medically unstable patient, is if there is a chance the procedure might be limited to a posterior-only correction. I believe that patients generally recover better if rehabilitation is not interrupted by a second operation, and timing for the second procedure can easily be affected by comorbidities. After a posterior-only procedure, I almost always brace the patient, usually for 3 months. I am much less strict about bracing after an anterior and posterior fusion.

Rotational injuries demand a similar strategy, with initial reduction, decompression, and stabilization posteriorly. These injuries are highly unstable and should be considered for anterior fixation as well. When this is not possible or practical, posterior constructs alone with pedicle screws and crosslinks can provide very stable fixation.[26] If fixation of these injuries is limited to a posterior procedure, most often because of significant comorbidities, I usually fuse two to three levels above and below for better control. This approach has achieved good long-term maintenance of correction in a limited number of patients. These patients all happened to have significant spinal cord injuries as well. I brace these patients for a minimum of 3 months and follow them closely during the initial postoperative period.

In patients without neurologic injury, the decision is less straightforward. At my institution, we treat most compression burst fractures (type A) nonsurgically.[27,28] Some authors suggest that fractures with 50% canal compromise or 50% loss of height can be considered unstable, but I do not adhere to this strictly. Many type A fractures that exceed this deformity can be treated successfully without surgery. Some of the criteria I use for recommending surgery include the principles White and Panjabi[29] have defined; that is, the patient demonstrates a progressive deformity on a weight-bearing radiograph compared with a supine radiograph; the patient has neurologic symptoms; or the patient has so much pain that getting out of bed without a brace is impossible. Some patients are not braceable, or there is significant concern regarding compliance with bracing. Finally, in the patient with multiple injuries who cannot wear a brace or who needs better stabilization to mobilize effectively, I believe a short segment fusion is justified.

I almost always approach compression burst fractures from the back using short segment fusion. Dick[30] and Gertzbein and associates[31] suggest that to obtain an effective reduction, the posterior procedure should be done within 4 to 5 days, and some suggest even longer. Because the effectiveness of ligamentotaxis diminishes progressively with time, however, I recommend performing the surgery within 1 to 2 days if possible for optimal results. Although the magnitude of the deformity, within certain limits, does not necessarily correlate with the success of the functional outcome, once I have a patient in surgery, I attempt to correct the deformity as much as possible. In addition, early surgery allows early mobilization. When surgery must be delayed for several days, in most cases I still approach it posteriorly and correct as much as possible, though I do not expect to achieve as much correction. If the delay is several weeks, the fracture is approached anteriorly. If severe comminution of the vertebral body is present and loss of correction and possibly fixation is a concern, an anterior procedure or longer posterior construct might be considered. I avoid anterior and posterior procedures in neurologically normal patients unless the vertebral body is extremely comminuted and the patient will not tolerate bracing. Although not an approved indication at this time, a carefully performed kyphoplasty using an injectable mineral bone cement (not polymethylmethacrylate) might be considered to avoid an anterior procedure but still provide anterior column support during the initial stages of healing. Again, this is appropriate only in the intact patient who does not require a decompression.

A distraction injury in a neurologically intact patient, on the other hand, is rarely managed nonsurgically. These injuries have a significant risk of progression, so I stabilize them, again with a posterior procedure. If the mechanical axis is such that there is no compression injury to the vertebral body, I simply reduce the injury with compression posteriorly with short segment pedicle screw fixation. If the axis causes vertebral body compression, some degree of anterior ligamentotaxis is achieved with lordosis of the instrumentation while the distraction injury is reduced posteriorly with compression. Care must be taken not to distract the fixation in an effort to obtain a better reduction anteriorly. Surgery is not indicated, however, for distraction injuries that propagate completely through the vertebral body and bony posterior elements with no ligamentous disruption. These are treated in a cast or brace initially and followed closely.

Rotational injuries are associated with a high rate of neurologic involvement. In patients with rotational injuries and no neurologic deficit, I stabilize initially from the back using short segment fixation. Depending on the magnitude of the injury, a longer posterior fusion or supplementary anterior fusion may be required as well. I try to make this decision preoperatively and, as long as the patient can tolerate it, complete the front and back procedures in a single stage. Because these injuries tend to be quite unstable, if I am performing posterior surgery only, I generally fuse at least two levels above and below the injury. For an anterior and posterior procedure, fixation can be limited to one level above and below the injury.

REHABILITATION

With these injuries, the initial hospitalization is only the first stage of recovery. A comprehensive rehabilitation program is essential to optimize outcomes and minimize complications, particularly in patients with neurologic deficits. With proper management, most patients will be able to return to some meaningful form of employment.

COMPLICATIONS

Complications were discussed at length in chapter 13, but I will repeat a few general ideas. The physical examination should be conducted very diligently, looking carefully for associated injuries, as they are common. Spine fractures hurt, and pain control is important to facilitate mobilization. Neuropathic pain can be extremely difficult to control. Given the combination of trauma, pain medicine, and immobility, an ileus can be expected. The patient's diet should be controlled initially, and early mobilization is important. Skin care is also very important because pressure ulcers can be one of the biggest obstacles to rehabilitation. Finally, for deep venous thrombosis prophylaxis, I use antiembolism stockings and sequential compression devices in all patients until they are up and moving consistently. In patients with spinal cord injury, I use pharmacologic prophylaxis as well. The time this is started varies, depending on other injuries, the amount of epidural bleeding present during surgery, and underlying medical conditions. The use of filters can be very helpful in high-risk patients.[32] Recently, removable filters have become an option as well.

CONCLUSION

Optimal management of thoracolumbar fractures depends on many aspects of care. Proper and expeditious assessment and stabilization minimize initial deterioration. An understanding of biomechanics and a thorough physical examination coupled with sophisticated imaging provide the basis for deciding between surgical and non-surgical treatment options. Various surgical techniques can be used, as long as certain goals are met regarding decompression and/or stabilization. Advances in surgical techniques and the advent of comprehensive rehabilitation centers have further improved outcomes in patients with unstable thoracolumbar fractures. Continuing investigations into the biomechanics of these injuries as well as neurologic protection and repair promise to yield information that will further minimize risks and improve the management and outcomes of these injuries.

REFERENCES

1. Rhee PM, Bridgeman A, Acosta JA, et al: Lumbar fractures in adult blunt trauma: Axial and single-slice helical abdominal and pelvic computed tomographic scans versus portable plain films. *J Trauma* 2002;53:663-667.

2. Keenen TL, Antony J, Benson DR: Non-contiguous spinal fractures. *J Trauma* 1990;30:489-491.

3. Campbell SE, Phillips CD, Dubovsky E, Cail WS, Omary RA: The value of CT in determining potential instability of simple wedge-compression fractures of the lumbar spine. *AJNR Am J Neuroradiol* 1995;16:1385-1392.

4. Krueger MA, Green DA, Hoyt D, Garfin SR: Overlooked spine injuries associated with lumbar transverse process fractures. *Clin Orthop* 1996;327:191-195.

5. Pasquale M, Fabian TC: Practice management guidelines for trauma from the Eastern Association for the Surgery of Trauma. *J Trauma* 1998;44:941-956.

6. Gestring ML, Gracias VH, Feliciano MA, et al: Evaluation of the lower spine after blunt trauma using abdominal computed tomographic scanning supplemented with lateral scanograms. *J Trauma* 2002;53:9-14.

7. Blackmore CC, Ramsey SD, Mann FA, Deyo RA: Cervical spine screening with CT in trauma patients: A cost-effectiveness analysis. *Radiology* 1999;212:117-125.

8. Rybicki F, Nawfel RD, Judy PF, et al: Skin and thyroid dosimetry in cervical spine screening: Two methods for evaluation and a comparison between a helical CT and radiographic trauma series. *AJR Am J Roentgenol* 2002;179:933-937.

9. Bracken MB, Shepard MJ, Holford TR, et al: Methylprednisolone or tirilazad mesylate administration after acute spinal cord injury: 1-year follow up. Results of the third National Acute Spinal Cord Injury randomized controlled trial. *J Neurosurg* 1998;89:699-706.

10. Geisler FH, Coleman WP, Grieco G, Poonian D Sygen Study Group: The Sygen multicenter acute spinal cord injury study. *Spine* 2001;26(suppl):87-98.

11. Panjabi MM, Kifune M, Wen L, et al: Dynamic canal encroachment during thoracolumbar burst fractures. *J Spinal Disord* 1995;8:39-48.

12. Benzel EC, Larson SJ: Functional recovery after decompressive operation for thoracic and lumbar spine fractures. *Neurosurgery* 1986;19:772-778.

13. Bohlman HH, Kirkpatrick JS, Delamarter RB, Leventhal M: Anterior decompression for late pain and paralysis after fractures of the thoracolumbar spine. *Clin Orthop* 1994;300:24-29.

14. Gertzbein SD: Scoliosis Research Society. Multicenter spine fracture study. *Spine* 1992;17:528-540.

15. Delamarter RB, Sherman J, Carr JB: Pathophysiology of spinal cord injury: Recovery after immediate and delayed decompression. *J Bone Joint Surg Am* 1995;77:1042-1049.

16. Fehlings MG, Sekhon LH, Tator C: The role and timing of decompression in acute spinal cord injury: What do we know? What should we do? *Spine* 2001;26(suppl):101-110.

17. Vaccaro AR, Daugherty RJ, Sheehan TP, et al: Neurologic outcome of early versus late surgery for cervical spinal cord injury. *Spine* 1997;22:2609-2613.

18. McLain RF, Benson DR: Urgent surgical stabilization of spinal fractures in polytrauma patients. *Spine* 1999;24:1646-1654.

19. Bradford DS, McBride GG: Surgical management of thoracolumbar spine fractures with incomplete neurologic deficits. *Clin Orthop* 1987;218:201-216.

20. Esses SI, Botsford DJ, Kostuik JP: Evaluation of surgical treatment for burst fractures. *Spine* 1990;15:667-673.

21. Kaneda K, Taneichi H, Abumi K, Hashimoto T, Satoh S, Fujiya M: Anterior decompression and stabilization with the Kaneda device for thoracolumbar burst fractures associated with neurological deficits. *J Bone Joint Surg Am* 1997;79:69-83.

22. McLain RF, Sparling E, Benson DR: Early failure of short-segment pedicle instrumentation for thoracolumbar fractures: A preliminary report. *J Bone Joint Surg Am* 1993;75:162-167.

23. Chiba M, McLain RF, Yerby SA, Moseley TA, Smith TS, Benson DR: Short-segment pedicle instrumentation: Biomechanical analysis of supplemental hook fixation. *Spine* 1996;21:288-294.

24. McCormack T, Karaikovic E, Gaines RW: The load sharing classification of spine fractures. *Spine* 1994;19:1741-1744.

25. Parker JW, Lane JR, Karaikovic EE, Gaines RW: Successful short-segment instrumentation and fusion for thoracolumbar spine fractures: A consecutive 4 1/2-year series. *Spine* 2000;25:1157-1170.

26. Dick JC, Zdeblick TA, Bartel BD, Kunz DN: Mechanical evaluation of cross-link designs in rigid pedicle screw systems. *Spine* 1997;22:370-375.

27. Mumford J, Weinstein JN, Spratt KF, Goel VK: Thoracolumbar burst fractures: The clinical efficacy and outcome of nonoperative management. *Spine* 1993;18:955-970.

28. Wood K, Butterman G, Mehbod A, Garvey T, Jhanjee R, Sechriest V: Operative compared with nonoperative treatment of a thoracolumbar burst fracture without neurological deficit. A prospective, randomized study. *J Bone Joint Surg Am* 2003;85:773-781.

29. White AA, Panjabi MM: The problem of clinical instability in the human spine: A systematic approach, in White AA, Panjabi MM (eds): *Clinical Biomechanics of the Spine.* Philadelphia, PA, JB Lippincott, 1978, pp 191-196.

30. Dick W: The "fixateur interne" as a versatile implant for spine surgery. *Spine* 1987;12:882-900.

31. Gertzbein SD, Crowe PJ, Schwartz M, Rowed D: Canal clearance in burst fractures using the AO internal fixator. *Spine* 1992;17:558-560.

32. Maxwell RA, Chavarria-Aguilar M, Cockerham WT, et al: Routine prophylactic vena cava filtration is not indicated after acute spinal cord injury. *J Trauma* 2002;52:902-906.

Index

Page numbers with *f* indicate figures
Page numbers with *t* indicate tables

implant alternatives, 62-63

nonsurgical treatments, 52-53

osteoporotic fractures, 102-103

posterior management (thoracolumbar fractures), 75-78

postoperative management and rehabilitation, 113-117

spinal cord injuries, 43-45

thoracolumbar fractures, 84

Rehabilitation, 105-117, 132-133. *See also* Postoperative management and rehabilitation

Research findings, 9-10, 26, 50-52

biomechanics, 9-10

classification systems, 26

nonsurgical treatments, 50-52

Retained missile fragments, 92-93

Risk factors, 93-94, 119-128, 133. *See also* Complications and risk factors

Rotation (axial), 12

S

Screws (pedicle), 60-61

Secondary infections, 88

Second-stage surgeries, 68, 69-70, 69*f*

Segmental hook-rod methods, 60

Social and psychological systems assessments, 112-113

Spasticity, 109

Spinal canal compromise, 52

Spinal constructs, 58, 60*f*

Spinal cord injuries, 35-45

American Spinal Injury Association (ASIA) Impairment Scale, 38

anatomy, 36

classifications, 36-37, 38*f*

cauda equina syndrome, 37

complete spinal cord injuries, 36

conus medullaris syndrome, 37

incomplete spinal cord injuries, 36-37

evaluation and diagnoses, 38

incidence, 35

management (medical), 38-40

National Acute Spinal Cord Injury Study (NASCIS), 39-40

National Acute Spinal Cord Injury Study II (NASCIS II), 39-40

National Acute Spinal Cord Injury Study III (NASCIS III), 39-40

recommendations, 40

management (surgical), 40-43, 41*f*, 42*f*

indications, 40-42

instrumentation systems, 42

neural compression, 40-41, 41*f*, 42*f*

neurologic status, 40-41

nonemergent surgery timing, 42

patient-specific considerations, 42

spinal angulation, 42

spinal instability, 40-41

pathophysiology, 37-38

Stabilization (surgical), 69, 71*f*

Stable versus unstable injuries, 130-132

Surgical issues. *See also under individual topics*

anatomy (surgical), 1-7

anterior management (thoracolumbar fractures), 80-82

complications and risk factors, 122-128

anterior treatments, 124-125

posterior treatments, 122-124

decision making, 80-82

spinal cord injuries, 40-43

surgical management (implant alternatives), 55-63

anterior approaches, 61-62

anterior bone-implant interfaces, 57-58, 59*f*

Cotrel-Dubousset method, 60

fixation principles, 55-56, 56*f*, 57*f*

Harrington rod instrumentation, 59-60

ISOLA method, 60

pedicle screw fixation, 60-61

posterior bone-implant interfaces, 56-57, 59*f*

posterior instrumentation systems, 58-62

segmental hook-rod methods, 60

spinal constructs, 58, 60*f*

Texas Scottish Rite Hospital method, 60

T

Target distances, 86

Target tissue properties, 86-87

Tears (dural), 119-120, 122

Technical issues (anterior management), 82-83

Texas Scottish Rite Hospital method, 60

Thoracic vertebrae, 1-2, 2*f*, 3*f*

Thoracolumbar fractures. *See also* Fractures

anterior management approach, 79-84

anatomy, 79

anterior decompression, 80-81, 82*f*

anterior instrumentation, 83

biomechanics, 81-82, 82*f*, 83*f*